Better Physical Fitness

Dr VAUGHAN THOMAS

Better Physical Fitness

KAYE & WARD · LONDON
in association with Methuen of Australia
and Methuen, New Zealand

First published in Great Britain by
Kaye & Ward Ltd
21 New Street, London EC2M 4NT
1979

ISBN 0 7182 1461 7

Set in VIP Palatino and
printed in Great Britain by Cox & Wyman Ltd,
London, Fakenham and Reading

Contents

Foreword

With a mother who wanted me to be a concert pianist and a father who wanted me to be a champion athlete, it was obvious that I was going to have to make an early choice. At fourteen, in fact, I won my first national title and that was it. My life was dedicated to fitness and sport, with music as a means of relaxation and pleasure.

Of the thirty years which followed I spent almost half as a member of the greatest bunch of supermen around – that is, the physical education instructors of the armed forces. After a few years at college, I then spent the other half of the thirty years as a member of the physical education profession.

For over twenty-five years (and for a few more, I hope) I competed in all kinds of national, European, World and Olympic championships. I have coached and advised world class sportsmen from a dozen sports – and studied, researched, taught and written about fitness and sport.

What a wonderful life! But not for everyone. More and more I am coming to realise that fitness *is* for everyone, and sport is for the poor performer as well as the champion. That is why I felt I had to write this book; out of gratitude to my family, friends and colleagues; out of hope for the millions of youngsters who might like to taste some of the joys I have experienced; and out of a genuine desire to help humanity to raise its levels of positive health.

I dedicate the book to all members of the Physical Education Association, and in particular to that tower of strength – its general secretary Mr Peter Sebastian.

August 1978 V.T.

1. Why Fitness?

The trouble with school is that the teachers each seem to have a picture in their mind of the perfect 'you', just like parents do. The fact that your ideal may be different from theirs doesn't stop them working away trying to turn you into something you may not want to be. They 'Know what's good for you'.

Physical education teachers are just the same. They work on the basis that you should grow up strong and healthy, and able to join in games and sports without making a fool of yourself. In fact, you should be just like they are, as far as they are concerned.

But these days, young people are increasingly asking themselves the question 'why?'. They no longer accept blindly that adults know best. And that goes for 'fitness' too. How can youngsters think fitness is important when so many of the adult population are fat, physically idle, chronic smokers who get out of breath just switching on the television?

What is Fitness?

First we have to know what we mean by fitness. A square peg doesn't *fit* a round hole, a certain rhythm doesn't *fit* the lyrics, an acquaintance isn't *fit* to be your friend. The word obviously can be used in many situations. Yet it still means the same thing – 'to have enough of the qualities which are needed for something'. In our case, the qualities we are concerned with are physical ones, and we can define physical fitness as:

'enough physical capacity to cope with the physical needs of life.'

Since each person's life is different, each has different physical needs, and each person's physical fitness is different. For a young person it is even more complicated, for two reasons. First, youngsters have the problem of growing. It is difficult for them to realise that the body they will possess as an adult is built during youth. Despite the fact that each baby inherits physical patterns from its parents, the food and activity it gets during childhood are even more important to physical development. So, some of the fitness a youngster develops is aimed at a future need to be a well developed adult.

The second reason is of an even longer term. The fitness developed during youth can affect the middle and later years of life. It is unusual for youngsters to be

7

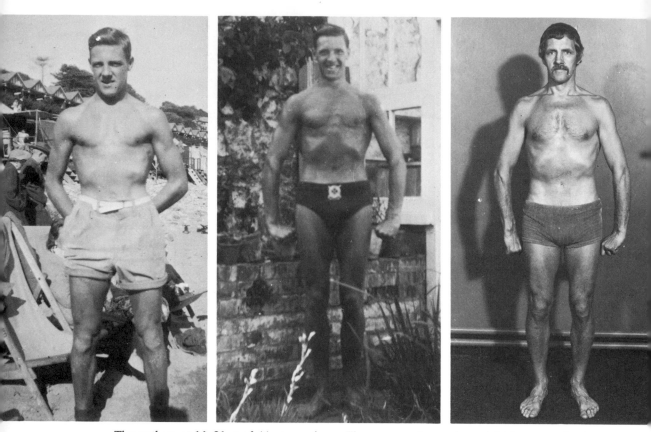

The author, at 16, 21, and 44 years of age. There was a change in weight between the first two from 158 to 170lbs. Between the second two – no difference.

concerned about these things; which is a pity. When you look at parents and grandparents, and hear them saying, 'I was like you when I was young', turn the statement round the other way. Do you want to be 'Just like them when you are old'? They may be wonderful people, kind, helpful, fun to be with. But they may also be physical wrecks slowly sinking in the sea of life!

So, we can see that there are three basic questions which must be answered:

1. How much fitness do I need to do the things I do now?
2. How tall, strong and agile do I want to be as an adult?
3. How long an active life do I want?

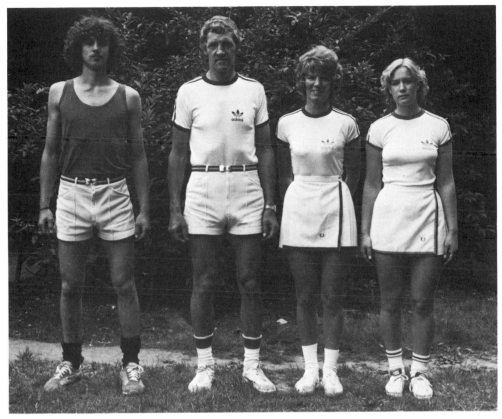

The author, his wife Christina, daughter Kim and son Garth.

Fit for What?

Physical fitness can be divided into four basic parts:

Strength
Suppleness
Speed
Stamina

Strength: This is the ability to exert a force on something; either to move it, to hold it still, or to control it while it is moving. You need strength to lift a bag, to ride a bike, to open a door – or even to switch on the television!

Suppleness: This involves being able to adapt the shape of our body to fit into a particular position, or to be able to change our shape without stiffness. Those with great suppleness make good dancers and gymnasts, while even gardeners and musicians need a lot of suppleness for some specific movements.

Speed: There are two parts to speed. The first is to be able to react quickly to something happening – like a starter's pistol, the amber traffic signal, the stumble on a stone. These are sometimes called reflexes. The second is the ability to move quickly, like running for a bus or throwing a cricket ball.

Stamina: Basically, this describes the ability to keep doing something for a relatively long time. It involves either being able to keep going without feeling tired, or despite feeling tired. Stamina also includes the ability to recover quickly from exhausting work.

There is a kind of general fitness, sometimes termed 'Positive Health'. General physical fitness caters for the variety of physical demands posed by ordinary life, and the maintenance of capacity until very old age. In a healthy society, everybody should have an acceptable level of general fitness.

Then there is a specific fitness. This depends on the specific physical activities you want to do. They may be soccer, cycling, gardening, mountaineering; or you may want to be a musician, shop assistant, miner, lorry driver or airline pilot. Many of the huge range of jobs and recreational activities people do need a certain amount of physical fitness. What most people do not realise is that the fitness they need is quite specific to the activity they need it for. A really fit athlete would find himself exhausted after a day's work as a shop assistant. A superstar badminton player would get cramp in his forearm muscles after a few minutes trying to play a violin. A house painter and a gardener would quickly earn themselves stiff muscles trying to do one another's jobs. A marathon runner is no good over a hundred metres. And so on.

We can see, then, that each individual needs some general fitness, and a sufficient amount of specific fitness.

General Fitness

Muscles. There are 215 pairs of muscles in the body which are called Skeletal Muscles. These are the ones which are fixed to your bones, and which cause movement. They also protect vital organs like the stomach, and cause the lungs to expand and contract, thus making you breathe. Another name for these muscles is Voluntary Muscles, because you can make them work by thinking about the

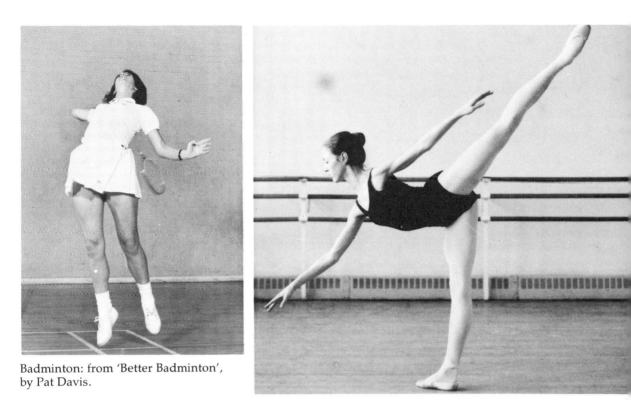

Badminton: from 'Better Badminton', by Pat Davis.

Ballet: from 'Better Ballet', by Richard Glasstone, photograph by Simon Rae Scott.

The fitness of a badminton player is very different from that of a ballet dancer.

movement you want them to do and sending them 'messages' to do it. This is what happens when a soccer player shoots for goal. Some of his skeletal muscles are holding him upright and keeping him balanced automatically, and some are being told by him what to do once he has worked out how hard and in what direction to swing his leg so that he kicks the ball properly.

There are other muscles which cannot be directly controlled. These keep the internal organs of the body working automatically, and include that most tireless of muscles – the heart itself. Since the heart never stops working for longer than a fraction of a second, and has to work harder whenever the body does any work, it is the most important item in general fitness.

Joints. Voluntary movement could not take place if we did not have movable joints. However, our movements can only really be controlled if the joints have 'safety belts' around them to stop them moving too far. These are strong straps of fibre called ligaments, and they need to be just long enough to protect the joint from dislocation.

Our movements can also be hampered by muscles being too tight. Bending over to put your palms on the floor, keeping your knees straight, will give you a demonstration of this. The muscles at the back of your thighs will probably prevent you from making it. Soccer players have problems doing this exercise because of their very strong and tight thigh muscles.

Summary. In general fitness, the main thing is to keep the heart in good shape. Whatever general work the body is doing, the muscles need extra blood to carry fuel and oxygen to the muscles. The heart pumps that blood. The fitness of the heart is a part of stamina, and whatever fitness training you do has *some* effect on the heart. There is also the important point that the heart needs to be fit to withstand the sudden physical emergencies which happen in life – causing heart failure in some people with weak hearts.

The muscles also need to be generally fit, which means *all* muscles. If your body has a particular muscle, it is because that muscle is needed; maybe not frequently, but if the muscle isn't in good condition it will let you down at that infrequent moment when you do need it. At times like that, stresses are put on other parts of the body like ligaments, cartilages or spinal discs. Literally hundreds of thousands of people suffer from slipped discs, arthritis, dodgy cartilages and the like just because their muscles weren't generally fit enough to withstand some stress or other.

In terms of general fitness, suppleness is not as important as many people make out. It may be nice to throw your body all over the place when dancing, but other than that too much suppleness can be a positive nuisance – or even dangerous. As long as you are supple enough to do the things you normally do, don't bother to develop any more suppleness. Keep those nice strong ligaments supporting your joints.

Specific Fitness

If there are specific things to do which need physical fitness, then that fitness will be developed to a certain extent by doing the activity. On the other hand, if you want to perform the activity better, or more easily, then the specific fitness needs to be developed apart from the activity itself. This process depends upon very careful identification of the specific muscles or joints which are being used, or the specific movement being performed. Not many people are very good at diagnosing specific fitness needs, though a good P.E. teacher or sport coach ought to be able to help. But in general it is very important to remember that the body movements and positions which are used in developing specific fitness should be identical or very similar to the movements used in the activity. For example, if the specific activity you are concerned with is skiing (like, you are going on a winter holiday), then you

need strength and stamina in the muscles of the front of the thigh *particularly in a crouched position*. Going for long runs won't do much good, whereas some 'squatting' exercises performed regularly for a few weeks will make the holiday much more successful.

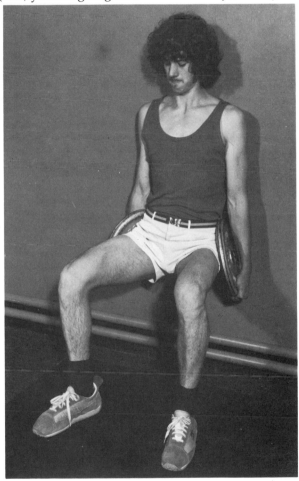

A good preparatory skiing exercise.

Feeling High

The best reason for being really fit, for having a high level of positive health, is the most difficult one to measure or to prove. Exercise scientists have pinned down all the easy things to measure about fitness; muscle A gains 10% in strength; heart X pumps 50% more blood; lungs Z shift twice as much air – all these things have been proved to benefit with fitness. In fact, some researchers have shown that people who are fit score better on intelligence tests, earn more money, or even have more sex appeal!

All these things are important, and exercise scientists are quite right to unearth the evidence to justify to people the need to be fit. On the other hand, of much more importance is the general feeling of being 'high'. The really fit person, particularly when generally fit, feels rather like a superman. The senses seem keener, nothing seems impossible, jobs are easier to tackle. Everything 'fits'.

The point about being high on fitness is that it is real and there are no unpleasant after affects. Alcohol and drugs are claimed to have this kind of effect, but it isn't real. Anyone who tries to do some supertrick when drunk ends up looking stupid, or injured. And the hangover!

Ask anyone who is really fit. They have answered the question for themselves. To look good, feel good, and stay that way for a long healthy life – those are the rewards of fitness.

2. Training

It is easy to talk about fitness. Many people spend a lifetime talking about it without doing much about getting fit. Many others spend a lot of time trying to get fit and failing. The clever ones get fit with the minimum of effort and fuss, and actually enjoy themselves while they're doing it.

Fitness is developed by doing exercise effectively. The process of doing effective exercise is called Training. It is possible to do exercise ineffectively, which is not training. There is a very simple principle on which training is based. *The human improves when given gradually increasing physical stress.* This is known as the Principle of Overload, and it applies just as much to the unfit exercise hater as to the Olympic champion.

Training must always start off easily. This applies to the first few of a long series of training sessions, but it also applies within each session. If the stress of exercise is too high, that is if the overload is too great, then something has to give way and an injury occurs. This happens a lot, particularly when someone is too keen (either the pupil or the teacher). An injury during training is bad news. It puts the injured person off doing any hard training in the future, and turns other people off as well. So don't be worried about what others may think in the early stages – take it easy and just go through the motions. Let your body get used to this new level of activity. It won't be long before it is crying out for more, whereas the idiot who rushed off madly at first will be sitting down nursing his aches and pains.

Once you are 'broken in', the level of exercise and the length of time you keep going can be gradually increased. Remember, your body is the best judge of the level of overload. Nobody pretends that intensive training is easy, and sometimes you have to push yourself very hard. But if your body says 'stop, you're damaging me', or if your aches and pains don't clear up by the next day, then your level of overload is too high. In fact, what is the point of rushing things – you have a lifetime in front of you.

Warm Up

In many ways the human is like an engine in a motor bike or a car. No one in his right mind revs. an engine hard before it has warmed up, it wouldn't be very long before the engine was a clapped out wreck. Exercise warm up is the same, and it means what it says. You should jog around, doing a few gentle stretching exercises like the ones described in chapter four, dressed in warm clothes like a tracksuit or sweater, until you feel warm and have perhaps begun to sweat. Then you should start the exercise immediately. There is no point in warming up only to cool down again before starting the training.

The warm up prepares you for hard exercise in many ways, but mainly it starts the heart beating faster, gets the muscles of deep breathing ready for work, and actually makes the voluntary muscles warmer and more elastic. It also has a psychological effect, stimulating your mind and most body systems ready for action, and shutting down the few systems which rest during exercise (like digestion, for example).

Apart from warm up helping you get the most out of your exercise, it is also very important in the prevention of minor injuries which can sometimes occur when exercising inefficiently. You may have noticed that valuable racehorses are always given a thorough warm up before a race. In this case, look after yourself as if you were a racehorse!

Warm Down

While it is common to see people warming up before exercise, it is far less common to see them warm down afterwards, even though it can be more important than warming up. Probably 'cool down' would be a better term, but it just isn't used. We have already seen that a human behaves like a machine, and most machines like to slow down gradually after running flat out. In your case, part of the process of exercise involves a build up of 'exhaust chemicals' in some areas of the body. If a gentle running and walking movement is kept going for a few minutes, with swinging and bending movements of the arms, the total recovery from the session will be much better.

Both warm up and warm down provide a good opportunity to have a chat with anyone involved in the training with you. Most people enjoy having company during exercise sessions, yet don't feel like talking – or haven't enough puff to talk – while pushing themselves to their limit. So, 'Talk Time' is before and after; and there is usually a lot to talk about.

The last and very important part of warm down is the 'clean up', that is to say, a bath. Apart from the great psychological value of the physical stimulus of a good bath following exercise, particularly a shower bath, a body on which large quantities of sweat have dried out begins to smell. This not only feels uncomfortable, but makes you much less attractive in close company!

The Fitness Curve

If you designed a training session for yourself, and used it every day for a few months without alteration, then two important things would happen.

First, you would get bored. Variety is certainly the spice of life in training, and is easy to achieve when you realise that there are thousands and thousands of different exercises in common use. More people give up exercise through boredom than any other reason.

Secondly you would find over the early stages that you made quite rapid gains of fitness, but as time went on those gains would get smaller and smaller until eventually improvement would stop. You would then be training just to maintain the level of fitness you had reached, which is called a 'plateau'.

Provided that you are satisfied with the level of your fitness plateau, that's fine. But, like a drug, the more you have of fitness the more you want – except that there are none of the bad side effects which occur with drugs! Training plateaux can be avoided by changing the exercise used, and by increasing the amount of effort put into the exercise.

If you manage to avoid the plateaux by these methods, then over a long time (maybe years) your fitness curve might look something like this –

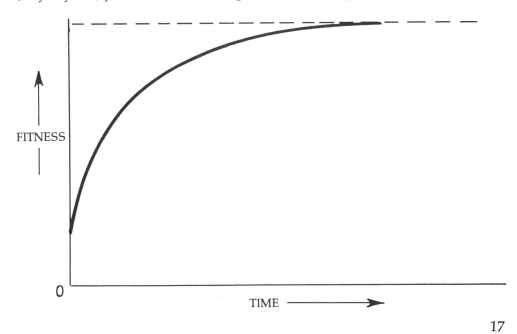

You would still reach a plateau, though at a far greater level of fitness than your early plateau. This represents the maximum development you are capable of, considering the amount of time and effort you can give to training. Of course, you may still continue to develop because you are still growing, and the training will still stimulate that development. But if by this final plateau stage you are an adult, then you will remain at this very high level of fitness provided you maintain the exercise. Some adults, and I am one, remain like this for the rest of their lives until old age inevitably and gradually slows them down.

Peaking

If you are training for something particular – it might be the school sports, a skiing holiday, or a vacation job on a farm – then you will want to reach a peak of fitness at the right time, just before the event. Some sportsmen and their coaches have got this off to a fine art, by peaking for the Olympics or World Championships. Even so, you can achieve the same kind of thing without such great precision.

All you need to do is to decide what kind of specific fitness you need, and how much of it. Then, work out your approximate fitness curve and see if it will be good enough for your purpose. If not then you must train harder, or longer, or with different exercises, or a combination of the three. All this sounds rather scientific, and it can be very precise at the superathlete level. But it needn't be too difficult for you, and in chapter seven there are some hints which will help, as regards monitoring your progress.

Overtraining

It is possible to exercise too hard. Without doubt, a superfit sportsman can drive himself to absolute exhaustion day in and day out without fear of harming himself. On the other hand there is evidence to show that some youngsters who over exercise, and this means three or four hours of hard work per day, begin to get 'run down' in medical terms. Also, the fact that bones do not fully harden until after school leaving age means that youngsters should be wary of putting stresses on bones which might deform them. These are real dangers of overtraining.

The kind of training sessions which are described in this book will not lead to overtraining. They are not intended to be performed for more than an hour in any day, and much less than an hour in most cases. Also, the lifting of very heavy weights is not encouraged by those who are not fully physically matured. Of course, some juniors do compete in weightlifting competitions for example. They will have been very carefully coached in the techniques of weightlifting, which reduces the risk, but there are many experts who believe it is wrong for them to compete at all at that age.

I must also stress that it is possible to keep very fit merely by playing strenuous games for an average of one to two hours a day; that is mainly how I keep fit now. But – I did the exercises when I was young, and keeping fit is easier than getting fit!

Organisation

Like any other job, proper organisation of your training will ensure that you get the greatest benefits in the minimum amount of time and effort. Too many people just casually turn up for training with only a hazy idea of what they want to do. They can easily have their training dictated by someone else who is training near by and just follow the more organised person – even if that schedule was no use at all. They waste time during the session wondering what to do next, fiddling around with equipment which has not been properly prepared, and maybe even injuring themselves by doing something at the wrong time, in the wrong place, or in the wrong way.

There are a few things which must be carefully organised; you can remember them by the word POCKETS.

Place of exercise; have you booked it, will it be open?

Other people involved; do they know, are they organised?

Content; have you planned the content of your session to fit the overall plan?

Kit; is everything in your bag, is it serviceable?

Equipment; is the equipment available, suitable, prepared, serviceable?

Time; are you sure of the time and likely duration of the session?

Safety; are you using the right equipment, methods, precautions?

Before any training session, it takes only a few seconds to mentally check POCKETS, yet it can increase the effectiveness of your training enormously. Anyone who has turned up for training having forgotten to bring his shoes, or to find the gym closed, will know the feeling.

Facilities

Many people are surprised to find how little is really necessary in the way of training facilities. Of course, most would like really super glossy facilities with every modern convenience and training aid. But that is just icing on the cake. The muscles which are working don't really know (or care) whether you are in a training place or a back shed, an Olympic stadium or derelict land. Many of the finest and fittest physiques in the world have been developed in backstreet slums, prison camps, jungle villages and the like.

In fact, a lot of people spend so much time and money travelling to train in super facilities that they get fed up and broke in the process. So they give up. It is important to distinguish between *competing* in the best facilities (if you are a competitor), and *fitness training* for that competition. Have a good look around you. Do you have a large garden, a spare room, a park near by, access to facilities at school? Can you make your own equipment from boxes, old furniture, bricks, household items? Ingenuity is a useful talent when planning training facilities.

If you do need access to facilities belonging to some institution or other (church, army, college, private home, firm) don't be afraid to ask. If what you are doing is worthwhile, and if there are a small group of you organised to do it, public spirited people will often do their utmost to help you.

Needless to say, facilities need to be looked after. A little care while you are training can save a lot of work and maybe unpleasantness later on. Training is something you will probably want to keep doing for years and years. If you abuse your facilities, you will gradually reach the stage of having nowhere to train.

Diet

A lot of nonsense is talked about diet. In developed Western countries the normal diet contains everything you need in order to develop a reasonable level of fitness. In fact, the problem is that there is just too much of things and people tend to get too fat, high blood pressure, clogged up arteries and so on. There is no point in becoming a food fanatic. Let your bathroom scales be your guide.

During youth, you should expect your weight to increase gradually most of the time, but sometimes quite quickly. This is a normal pattern of growth. Your weighing machine can confirm this rate of growth, which should be fairly similar to your gains in height until you reach a maximum height. Then your weight will continue to increase as you fill out to your final basic shape.

Of course, there may be hiccoughs in the growth curve at various points. None of us are absolutely normal. On the other hand, there are many children and youths whose growth curve strays consistently on the side of being overweight. The best indication of this kind of overweight is to take a pinch of flesh between thumb and forefinger at a point halfway between your navel and your hip bone. If that fat fold, as it is called, is larger than a centimetre then you are overweight.

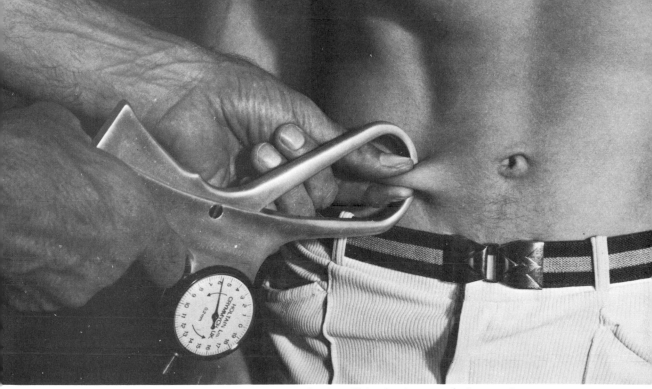

Garth has 0.58cm. fat fold, whereas Kim who is still in the 'puppy fat' stage has 1.6cm. despite being a very keen sportswoman.

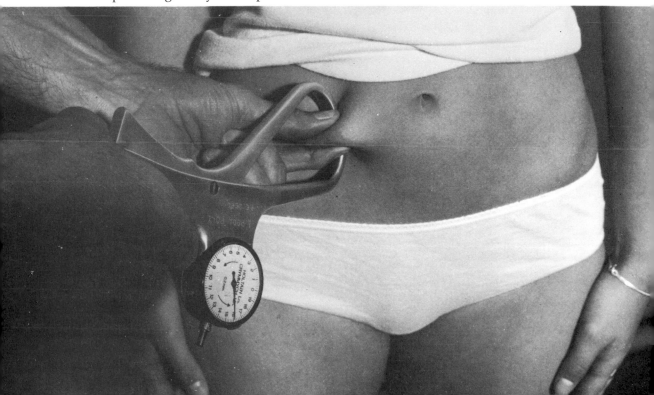

Mild overweight in youngsters may not be too serious, even though it means that they are not as fit as they côuld be. In fact, with girls it is quite normal to go through a 'puppy fat' stage where their shape is nothing like what it will eventually be. But whatever the cause a slight reduction in diet, particularly of high calorie foods, can usually keep weight within healthy limits. Your doctor, or physical education teacher, should be able to advise you if you think you are overweight.

Drugs

Since this book is concerned only with better physical fitness, it makes no moral judgements about drugs. In this case drugs are understood to be any substance which alters the way body mechanisms work and which are basically addictive. Included are drugs such as heroin, cocaine, LSD, marijuana; and also caffeine, alcohol and nicotine.

By their definition these drugs are potentially extremely harmful – even lethal. Some of course are less harmful than others, and can be tolerated by a very fit person in small quantities. There are no hard and fast rules, each person being unique in his reaction to drugs and fitness, except to say that *perfect* physical fitness cannot be achieved whilst drugs of any type are being taken. Having said that, each individual must reach his own compromise between being high on physical fitness and high on drugs. I personally value my own physical fitness far too much ever to take drugs other than caffeine and alcohol – and even these in moderation. The risks of taking any of the others are far too great.

3. Strength

Muscles can become strong in two ways – Quantity and Quality. Bigger muscles are usually stronger muscles. Competitive weightlifters are very strong, but their sport has to be divided into classes. Heavier men (who have more muscle) do not compete against lighter men (who have less muscle). So the quantity of muscle is important. Of course, some people want big muscles in order to look good. In their case, the muscles are stronger than normal, but because size is more important than strength, they are not usually of the same *quality* as a weightlifter's.

The methods of training strength all involve working the muscles against resistances. By steadily increasing overload, and the number of times each exercise is performed, the muscle gets bigger and stronger.

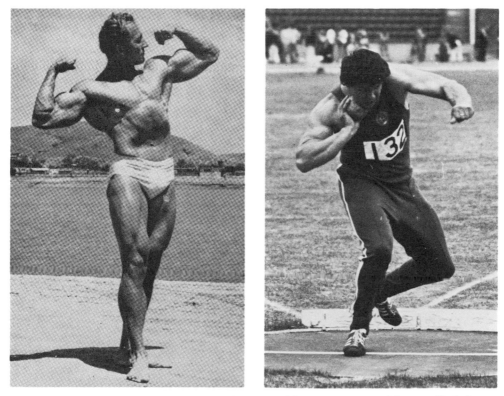

A bodybuilder wants good looking muscles – an athlete wants powerful ones. Each has a different kind of strength.

Definitions

There are some specialist terms used in training:

A Repetition – one complete exercise (abbreviated to 'rep').
A Set   – a number of reps of the same exercise done without stopping.
A Series   – a number of sets, with a rest between each.
A Session – a number of series of different or similar exercises.
Cheating – altering an exercise slightly to make it easier.
Load   – the amount of resistance to an exercise.

Resistance

There are many forms of resistance, including your own body, a partner, weights, springs, elastic materials, machines. The form of exercises can be static (where there is hardly any movement) or dynamic. Static exercises should be avoided whenever possible if they involve the trunk, and should never be done while

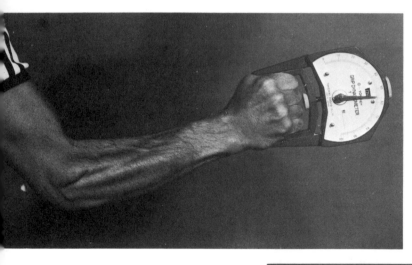

Grip strength difference between dominant (57kg.) and non dominant (50kg.) hands in well trained sportsman. Notice the difference in muscle development as well!

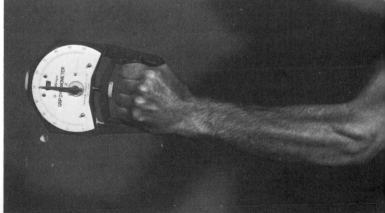

holding your breath. Otherwise, a great internal pressure is developed inside the chest, making it difficult for the heart to function properly.

Balance

It is normal for one side of your body to be stronger than the other. This is due to our habit of doing things usually with the dominant hand or leg. Our *natural* state, though, is to have a well balanced development. Any imbalance tends to create problems of posture, the way we hold ourselves – which can lead to arthritis in later life. Strength training should always be balanced, working just as much on each side either separately or together.

It is also common for people to be unbalanced in having stronger legs and weak arms, or vice versa; especially if they are training for a specific activity which needs strong legs *or* strong arms. In that case, imbalance may be very desirable, but normally it is better to have good all round strength.

Another case of imbalance is found when muscles causing one movement of a joint are stronger than the muscles opposing that movement. For example, if the muscles which bend the elbow (the biceps) are much stronger than those which straighten the elbow (the triceps), then the person walks around with bent elbows rather like a monkey!

A session ought to be balanced in itself, sets being rotated so that different body parts are exercised in turn, and different sides in turn. Careful thought on the balance of training makes a big difference to the value of sessions.

Reps and Load

For sheer strength, the load ought to be so great that only one or two reps are possible in each set. For size development, then lower loads and higher reps (up to about ten) are better. A well balanced series will start with low loads/high reps, continuing to increase the loads up to maximum. The series may stop there, or work back down to low loads/high reps.

Exercises

These are usually divided into arm, trunk (including neck), and leg exercises. Some common exercises will follow; only a small selection, but enough to start you off on your training programme. Although the exercises are grouped in categories for convenience, you will soon realise that most exercises affect several muscles and joints simultaneously.

25

Arm Exercises .

Handgrip   squeezing a tennis ball, large lump of clay, steel spring. Use all fingers and the thumb. Increase the resistance by using a newer ball, thicker clay, stronger spring.

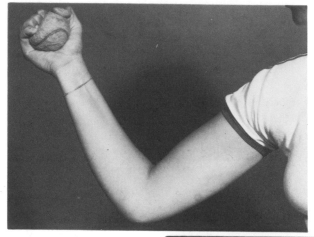

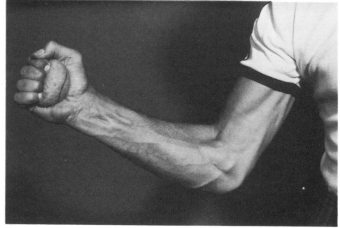

Wrist   wrist curls with barbell (palms down, and palms up) – can be done with single hand; or, firmly tie a weight via a 2 feet cord to a round stick of 2 ins diameter, then wind the weight up *and* down.

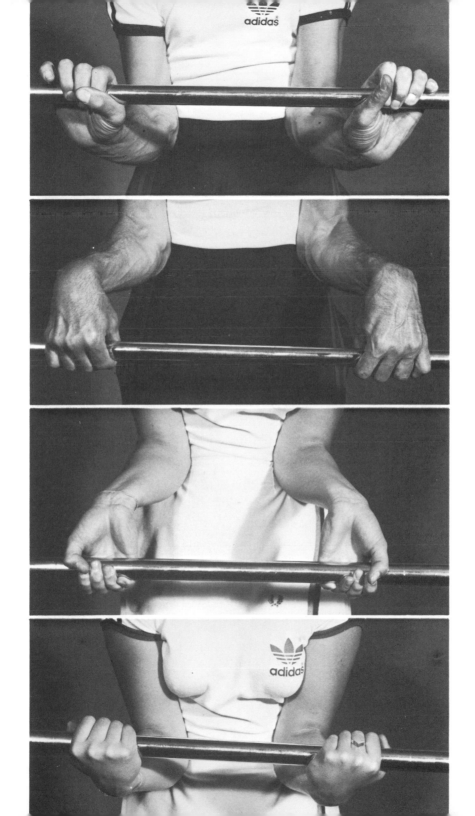

Elbow Bend   chins, either two hands or one; or inclined for girls (see pages 86 and 87 and description). Also barbell curls or springs where available.

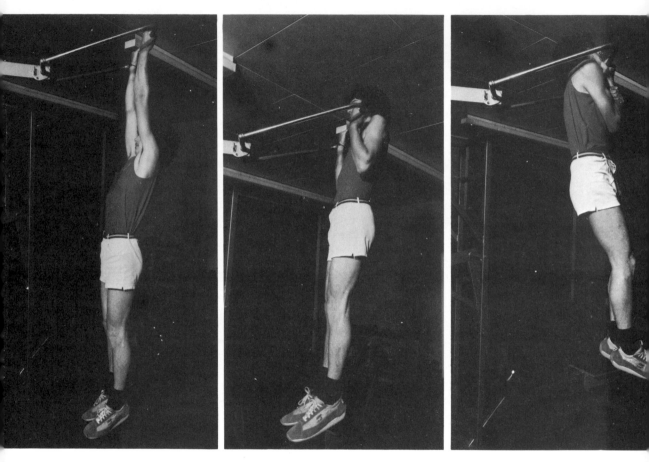

Elbow Stretch and Arm Push   press ups – straight forward, or inclined to increase or decrease the resistance. Keep the body straight, do not touch the floor other than with the hands and feet. Bench press – caution, adjust the machine or have an assistant if using a barbell, to ensure that the weight doesn't fall on you.

28

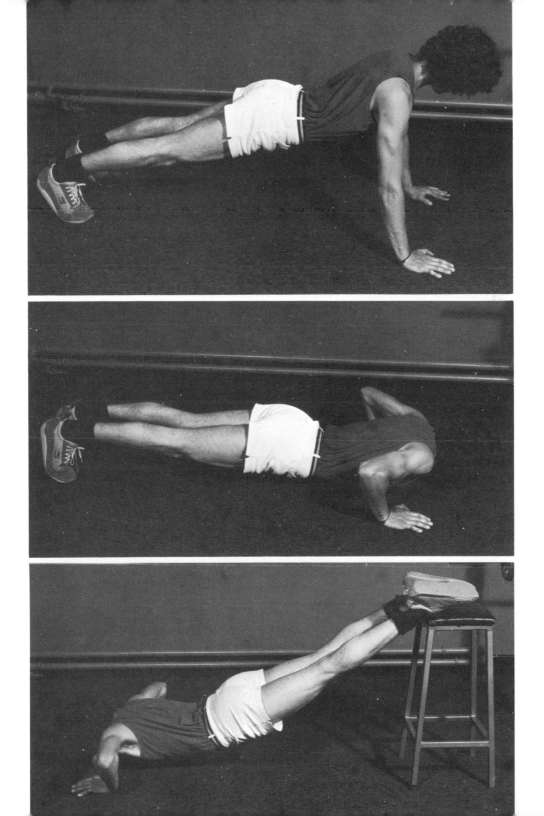

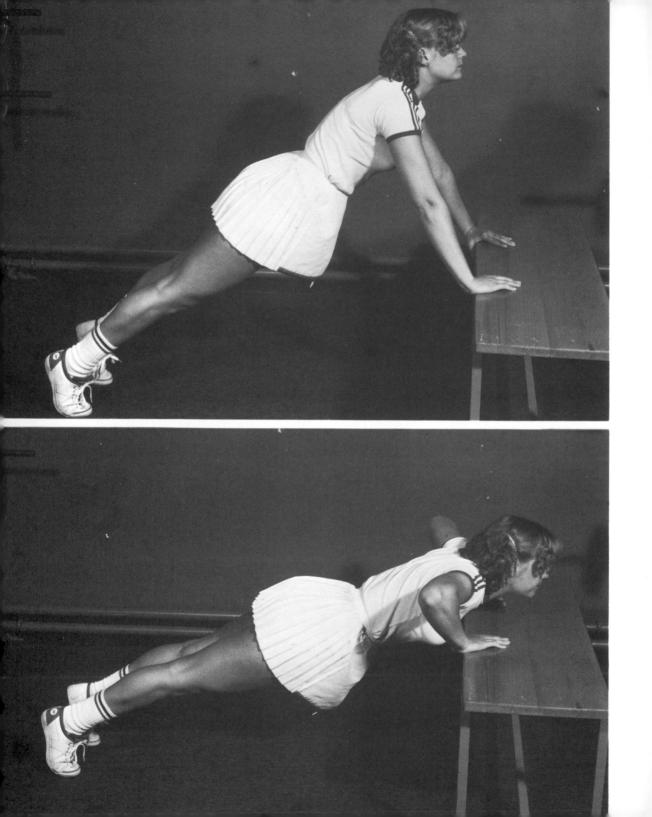

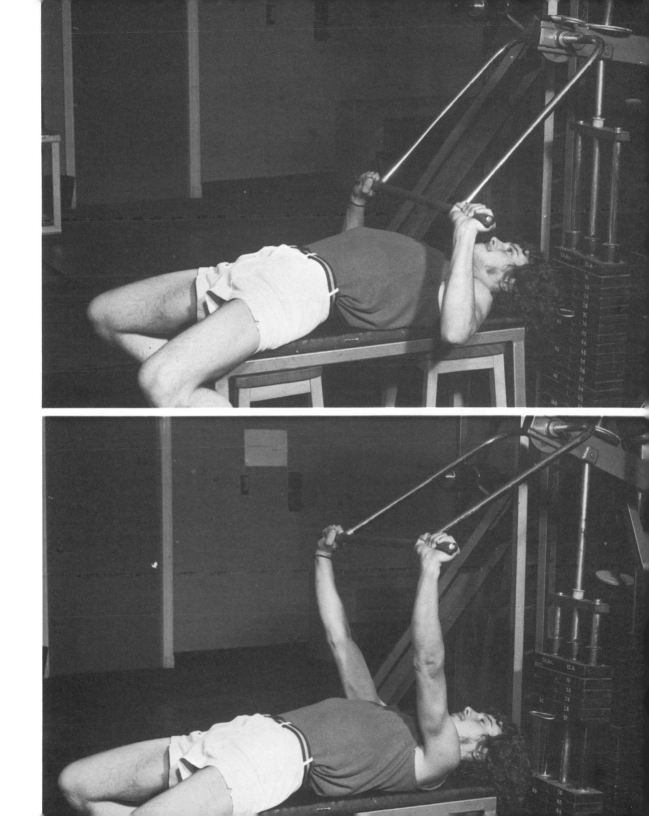

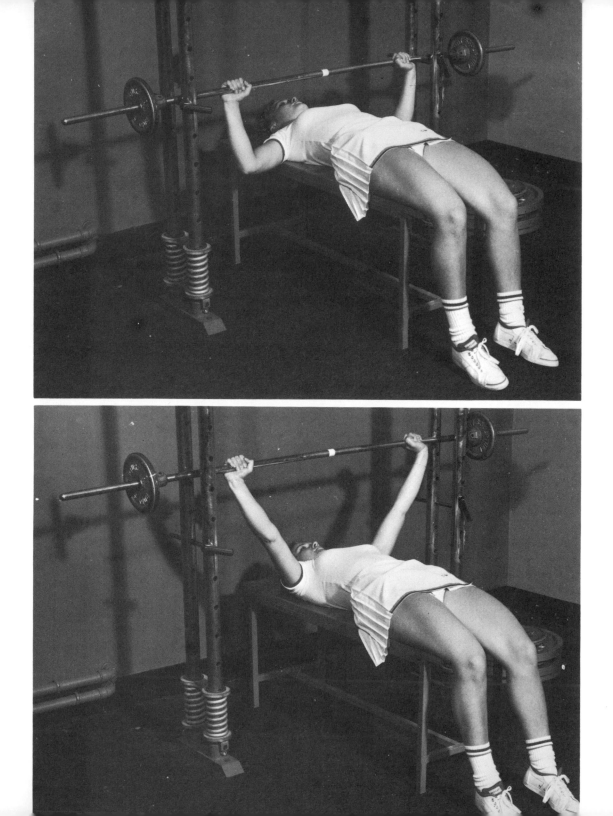

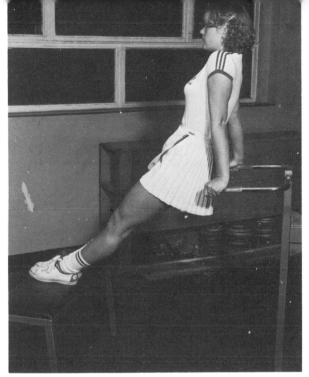

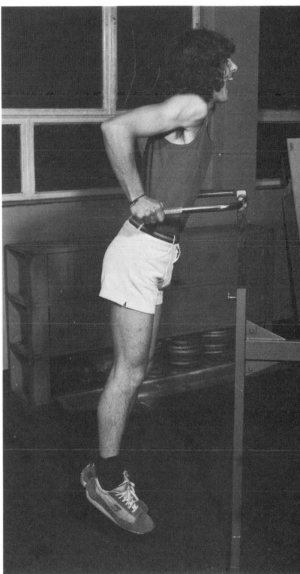

Elbow Stretch and Arm Lower dips – straight forward, or inclined to decrease the resistance. You should try to achieve a right angle at the elbow.

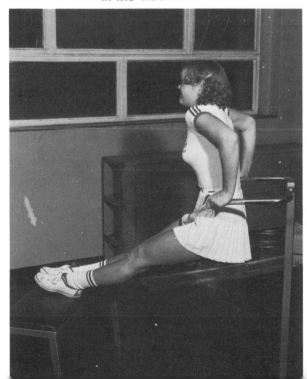

Elbow Bend and Arm Lower

lats – when you get really strong, you will need to hold yourself down with something heavy.

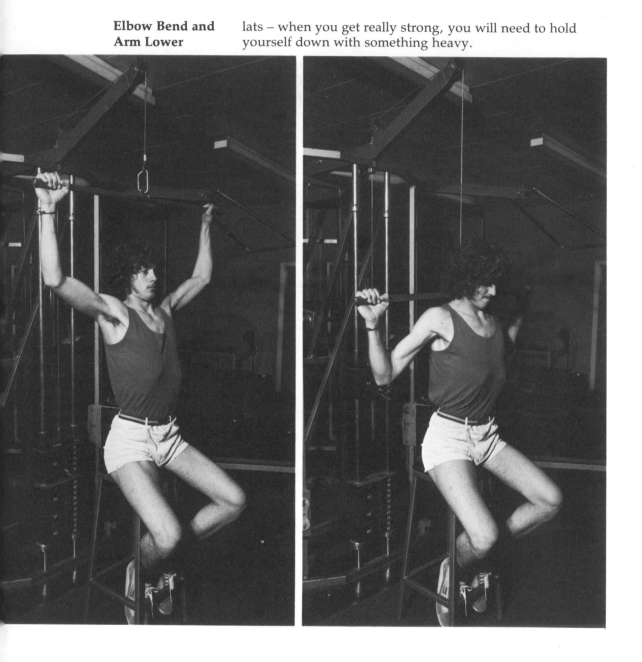

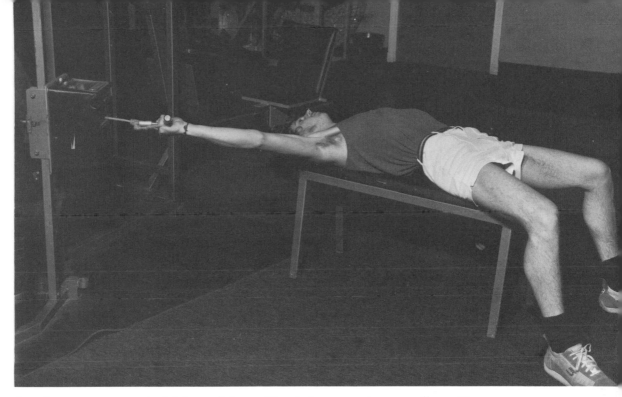

Arm Lower straight arm lats – with minigym, spring or pulleys. Keep arm parallel to floor as long as possible.

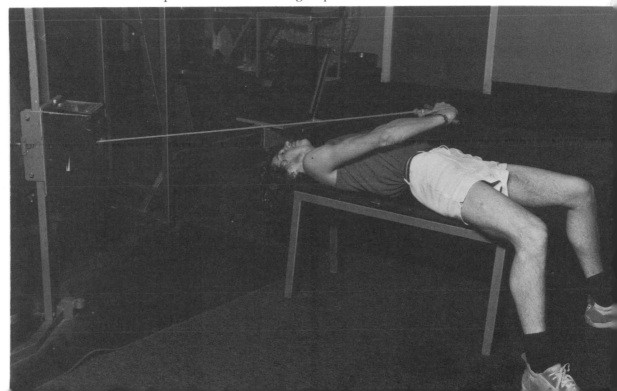

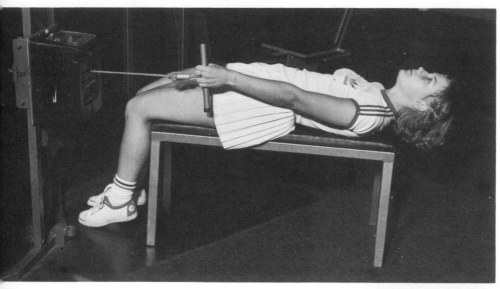

Arm Raise   straight arm
sideways raises –
with minigym,
springs, pulleys
or barbell.

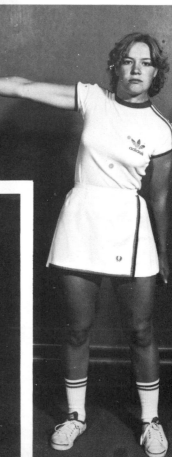

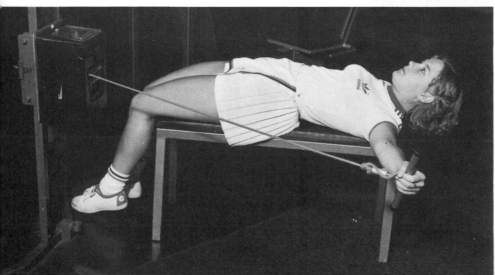

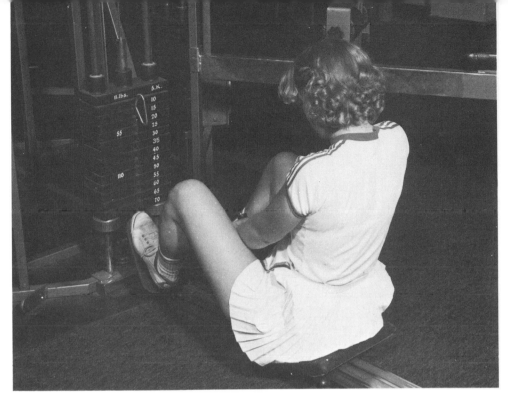

Arm Pull rowing (notice that done properly it is a back and leg exercise as well).

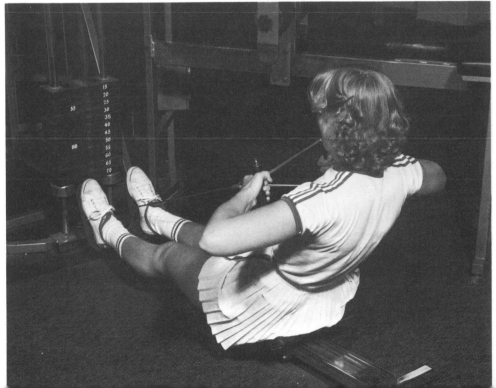

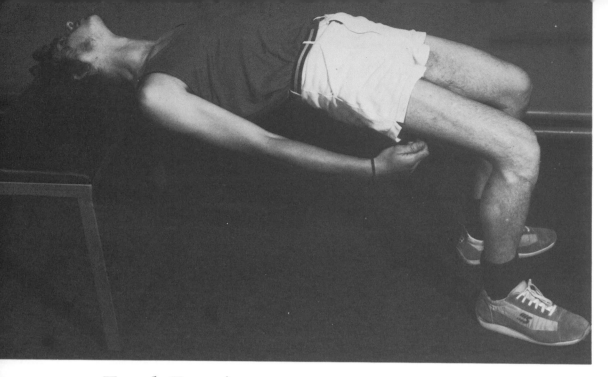

Trunk Exercises

Neck Rolling   unless you can obtain a head harness or special neck exerciser, you will have to use cushioned supports to do

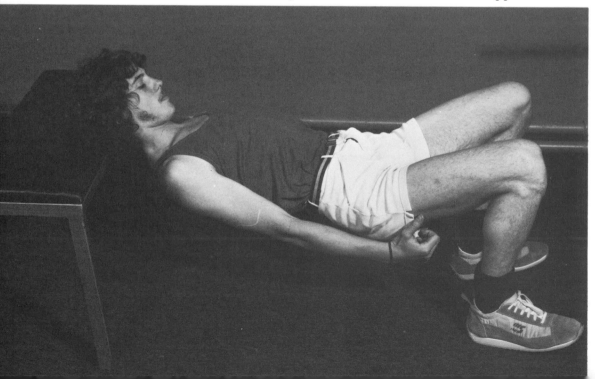

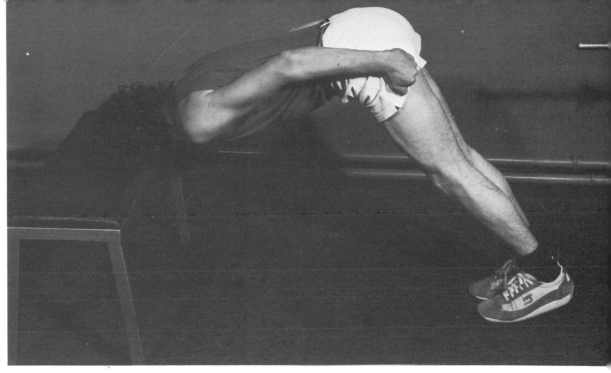

these exercises. They are very difficult, so work up to them gradually, taking some of the weight with your hands on the floor. Get as much movement in each position as you safely can.

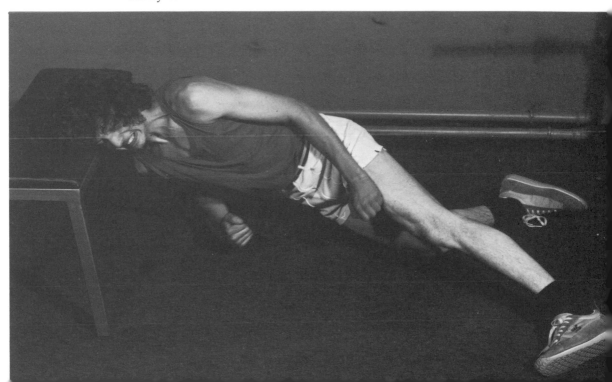

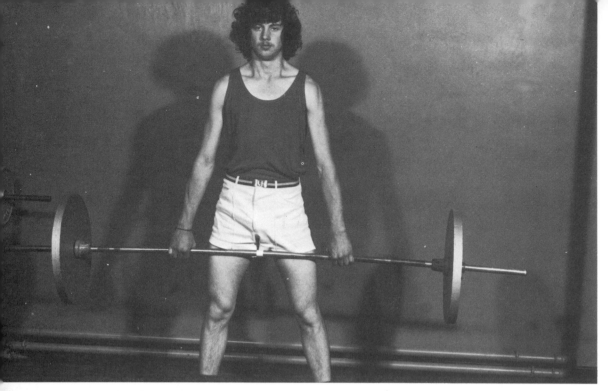

Shoulder Raise can be done with separate weights, try to get each shoulder to the same height.

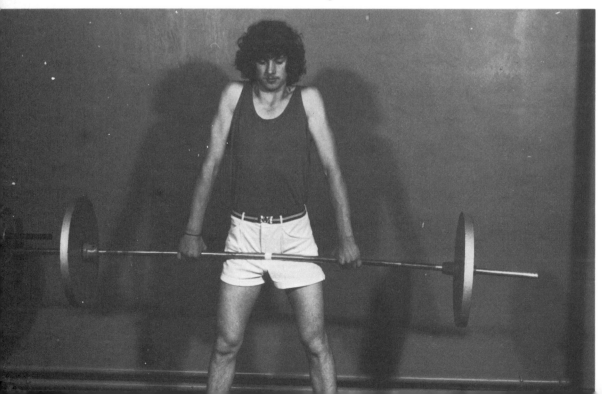

Shoulder Drop   lift your body as high as possible. Increase resistance with weighted belt, loaded rucsac, iron boots, etc.

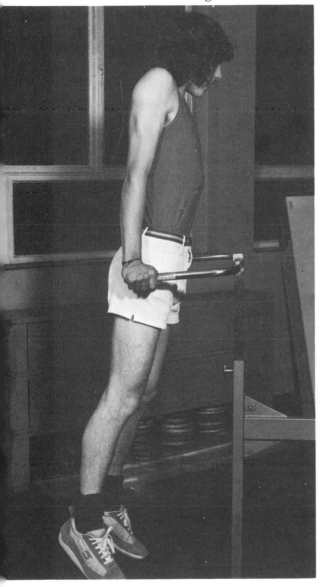 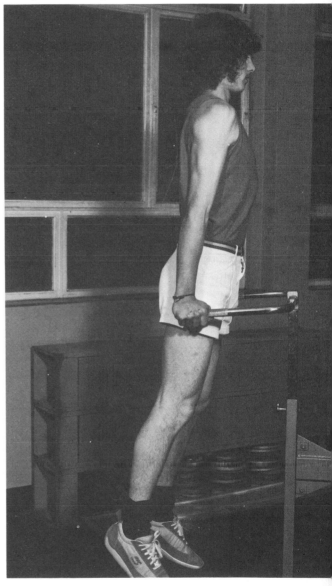

Chest Pulls   can be done with bent arms, also lying on the back with barbell, or springs, minigym and pulley.

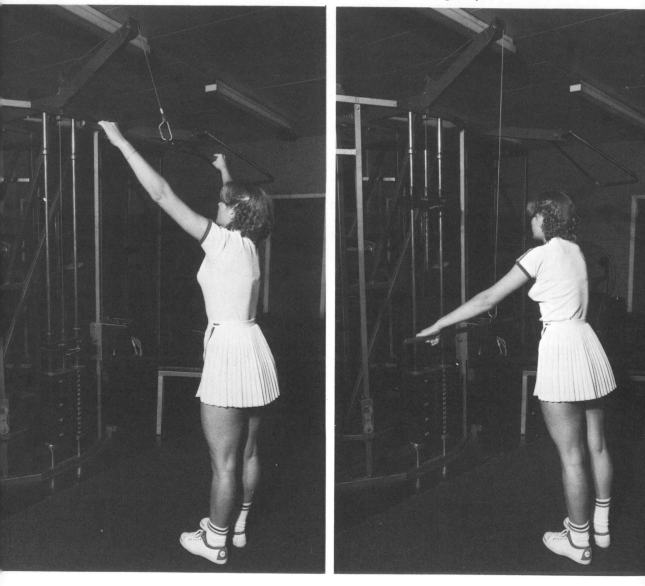

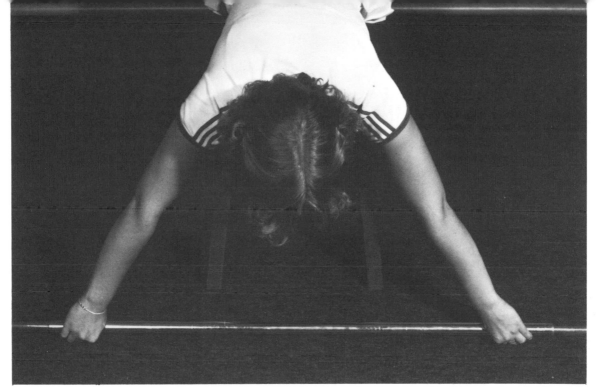

Back Pulls   this is such a weak movement that resistances are hardly necessary. The exercise shown is very difficult to do well.

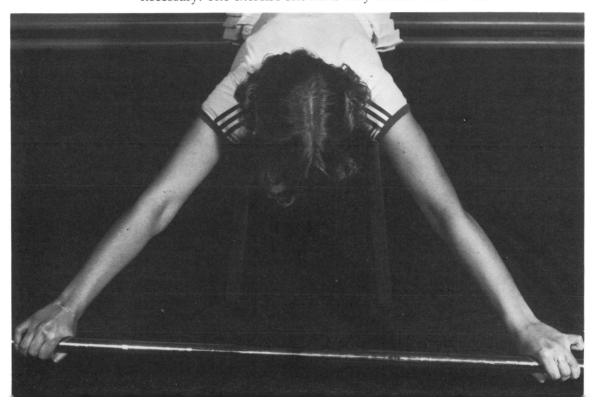

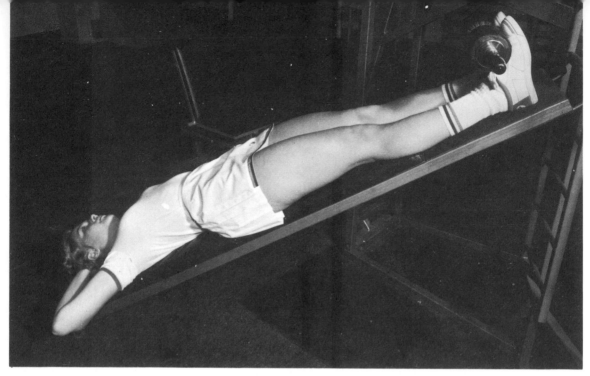

Trunk Bend   sit-ups – standard form shown on page 88: advanced forms shown here must only be done after much standard work first. Many other variations, including the use of weights.

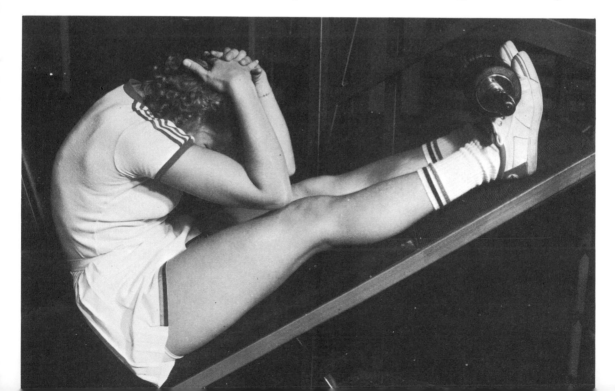

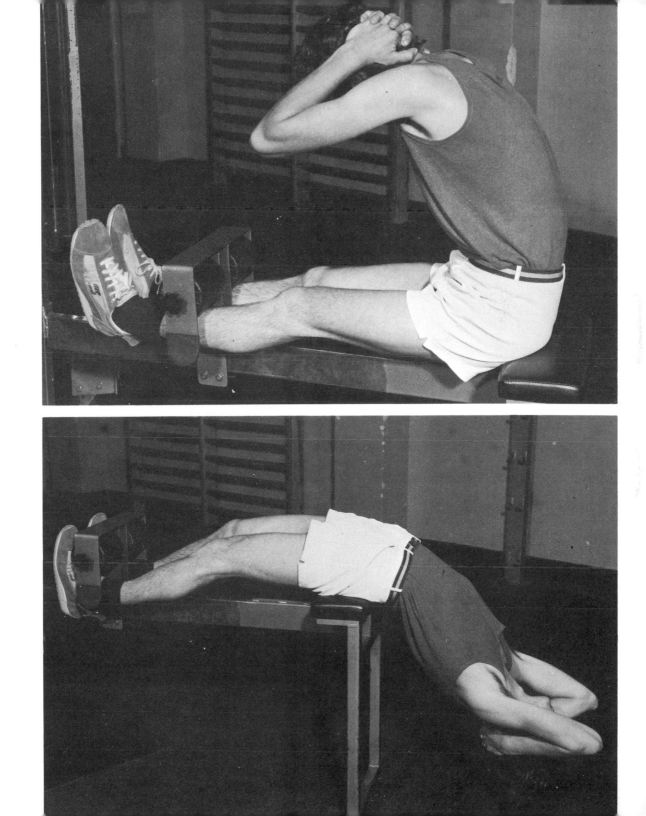

Trunk Stretch   back raises – again, a weak movement whose range can be increased with ingenuity or special equipment.

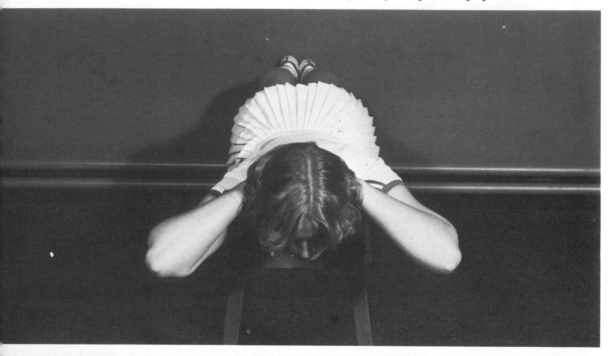

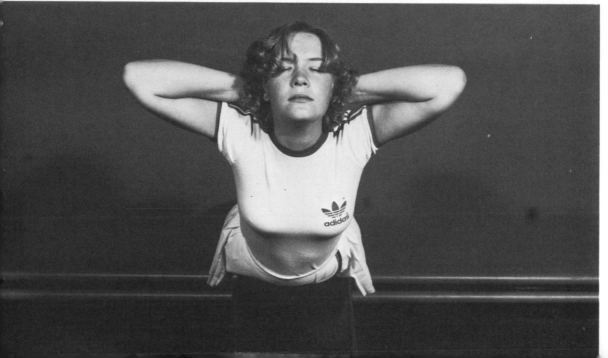

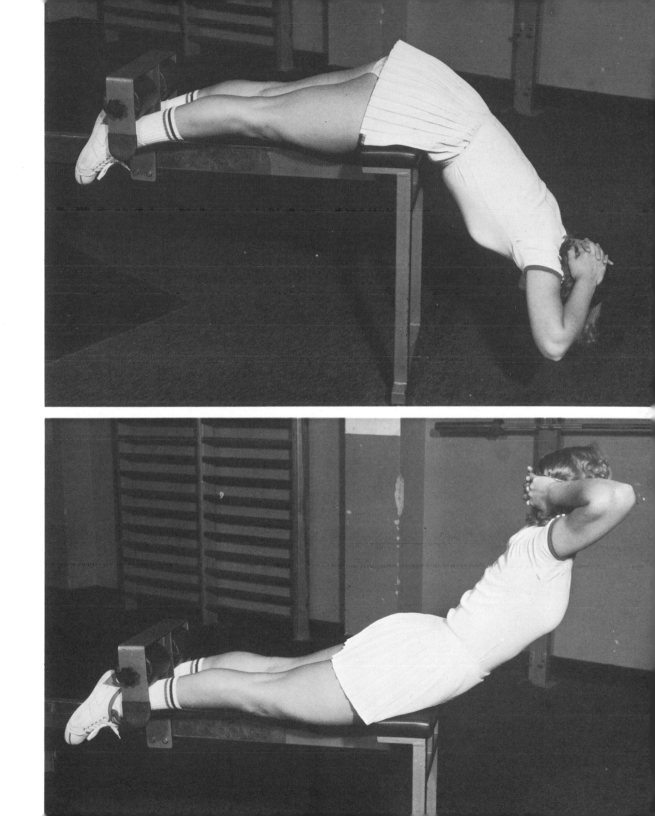

Leg Exercises

Hip – 4 ways   sometimes awkward to do. Keep leg straight, and wear an iron boot to increase the resistance.

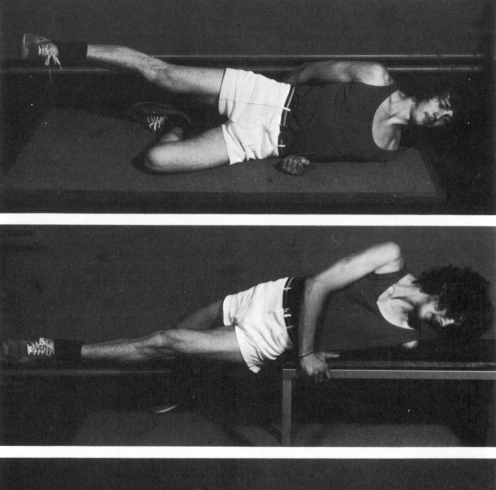

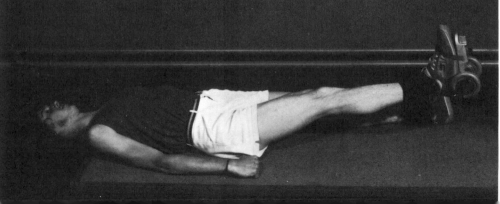

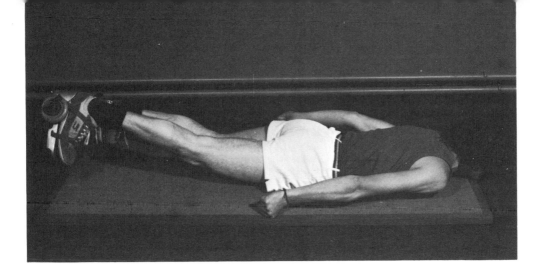

Knee Bend another awkward exercise – especially tough using the iron boot.

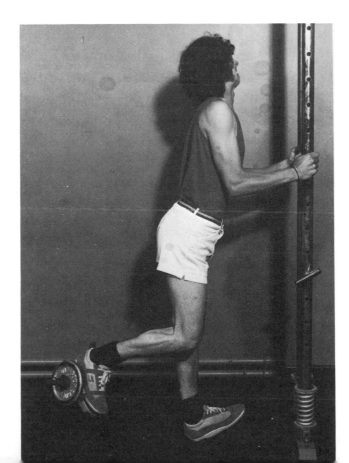

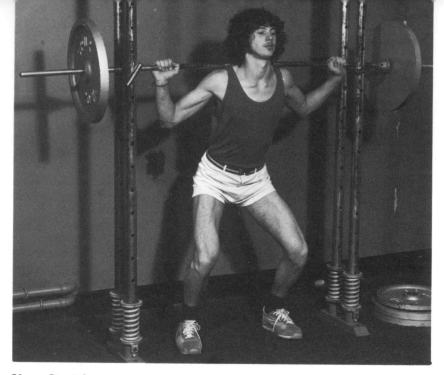

Knee Stretch squats – a firm favourite in many forms. Of vital importance never to go beyond a right angle at the knees, to keep the back straight, and to have assistance if not using a machine in case you collapse.

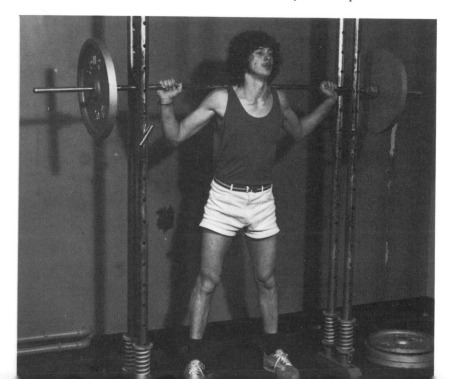

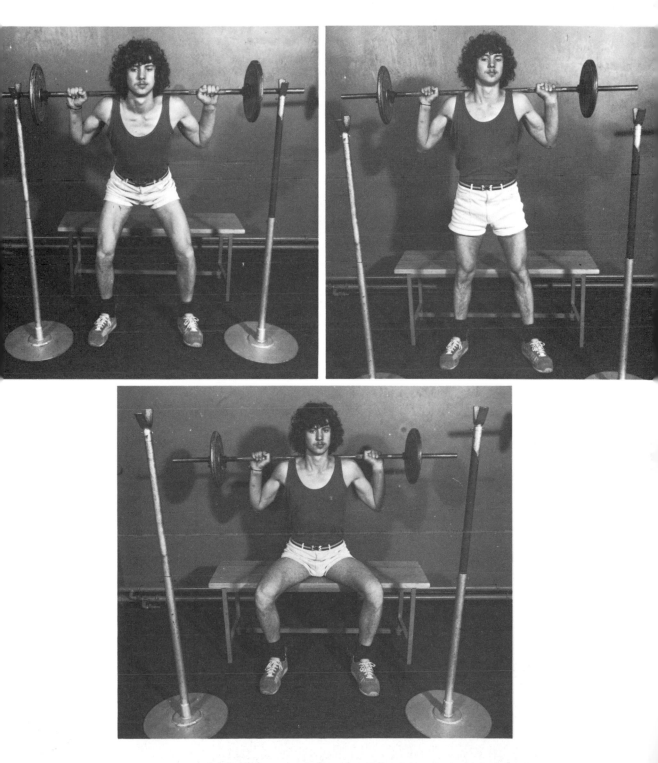

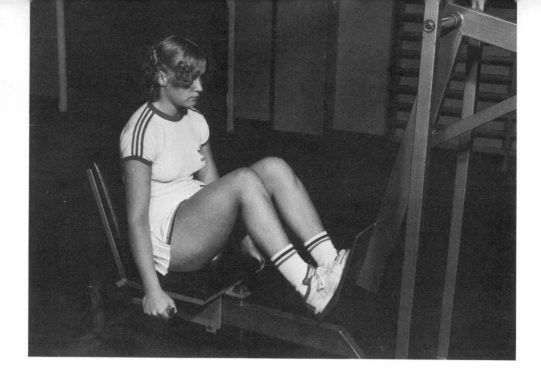

Knee and Hip Extend   leg press – facing up or down, one leg or two.

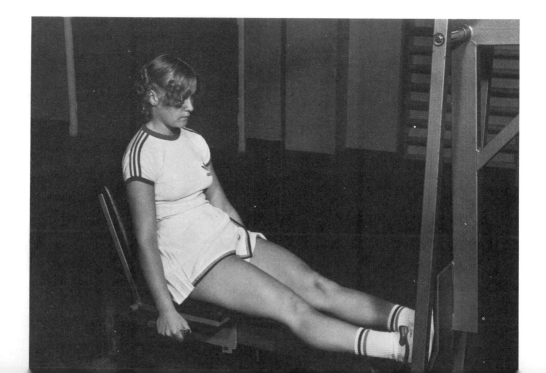

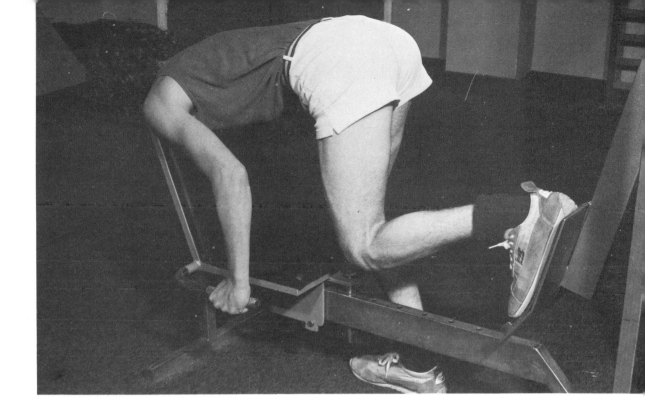

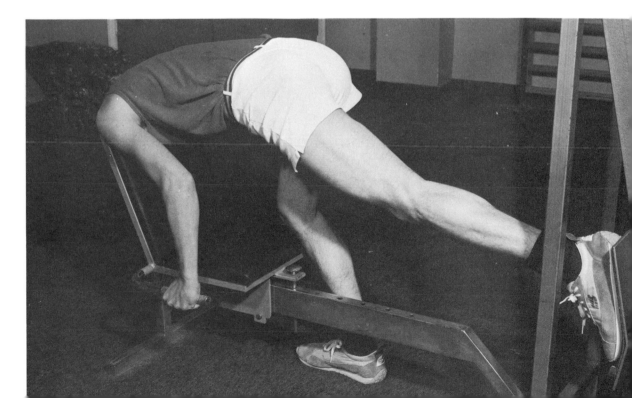

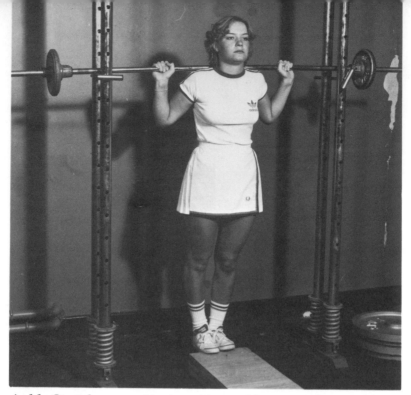

Ankle Stretch   calf raise with or without weights – ankle extensions using
the leg press machine. Ensure maximum range of movement.

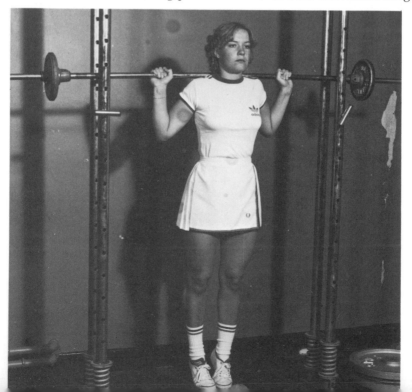

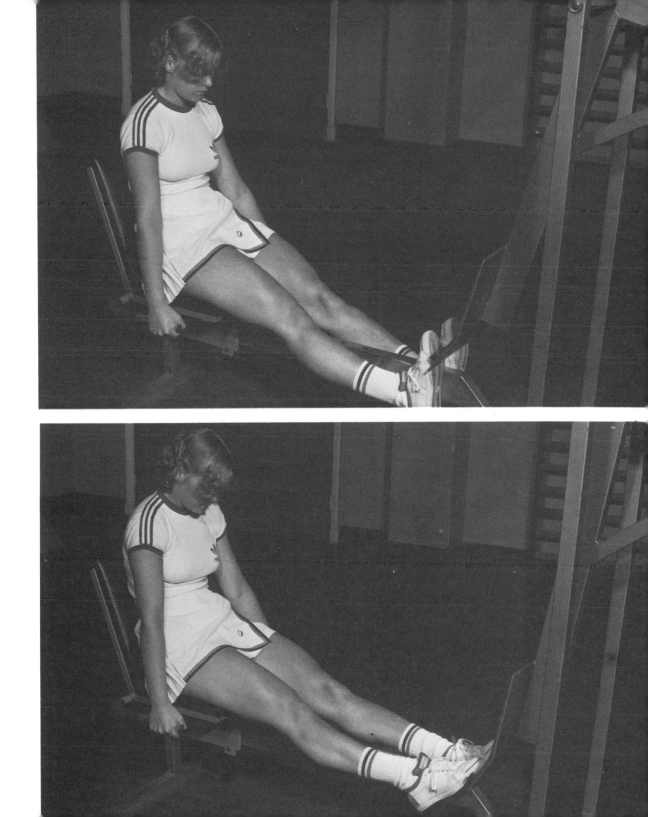

Ankle Bend difficult exercise to perform against resistance. One solution shown is to tie the bar on with your shoelaces!

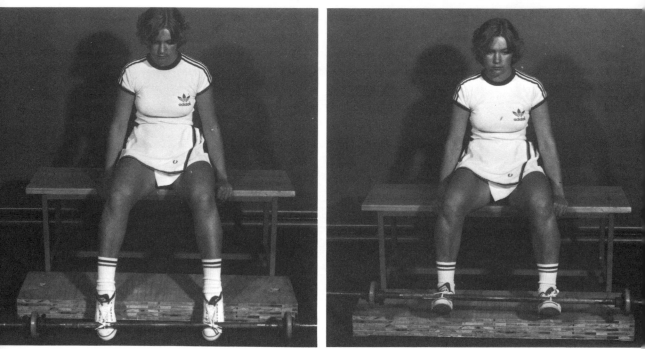

Tests of Strength

Of course, the best way to measure your own increasing strength is to measure the resistances you are working against. How much weight is on the bar; how many lifts can you do? On the other hand, apart from very carefully described competitive weightlifting movements, people tend to do these exercises in their own individual ways. So the performance of one person at an exercise cannot really be compared with the performance of another.

There are some well established tests, designed for people like you and used all over the world. If you test yourself with these every couple of months you will get an accurate idea not only of your own progress but also of how you rate against other people. You will find a couple of these tests in chapter 7.

4. Suppleness

In the introduction I made the point that you had to be very sure just how much suppleness you wanted. Too much can be as serious a problem as too little.

Just think about the way joints work. If you had no joints you would be absolutely rigid, and incapable of movement. On the other hand, if all your joints were absolutely loose, you would be permanently in danger of collapsing in a crumpled heap like an unsupported puppet!

This a diagram of a typical joint:

Capsular ligament   Synovial fluid

Synovial membrane   Hyaline cartilage

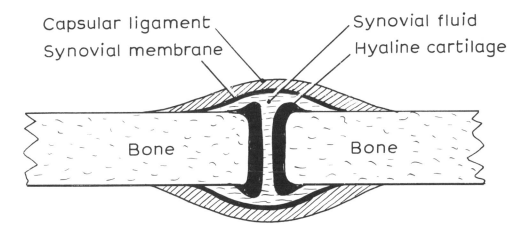

Bone   Bone

You can see that the joint is protected by its ligaments, which prevent bones from reaching extreme positions, and of course hold the bones together. If they become loose, the bones might get into positions where they are easily damaged. Particularly, the cartilage can become worn and torn, which leads to arthritis.

The joint is also protected by the muscles (and the muscle tendons) which act on it. If those muscles are strong then they can prevent a joint from getting into peculiar positions, or give it the support it needs when you really need to perform a very supple movement.

From this simple description of a joint, you can see that suppleness is developed in two ways: Firstly, by stretching or learning to relax the muscles which act on a joint; secondly, by stretching the ligaments in the joint.

The Muscles

Muscles are like elastic. They can be stretched, and then returned to their original length. As you get near the extreme stretching position, the muscle really resists being overstretched where, like elastic, it might snap or tear. For one thing, it sends you some warnings in the form of pain; but also it exerts a great force to resist the one which is causing the stretch. There is a limit, however, and any overstretching of the muscle will tear some of the muscle fibres. Great care must be taken to avoid this, the best guide being to avoid any sharp pains during stretching exercises. You must accept that there will be some dull pains or tight feelings when doing muscle stretching, in fact an absence of these means that you are not stretching far enough.

The Ligaments

Unlike muscles, ligaments are not elastic. When you flex a joint to an extreme position, if the movement is restricted by a definite obstruction with no feeling of muscle tightness or pain, then you can be fairly confident that ligament is the obstruction. In some cases the obstruction could be a bone, such as extension of the elbow joint, though strictly speaking ligaments still contribute to the restriction of the movement.

Ligaments should only be stretched very gradually. It may not be hard work, but it takes a long time. Any rush or overstretching will lead to ligament tears, which are generally slow to heal, and often lead to permanent weakness in the joint.

Methods of Stretching

Exercise specialists have always argued about the best ways of developing suppleness. One group thinks that vigorous bouncy movements are best, others feel that slow pressing actions are more effective. Some believe that passive work will do the trick, where the stretching force is applied by someone or something else. As usual, there is a little truth in all the methods, and pain is the only way for you to be sure that you are not being harmed by whatever method you are using. One point about being stretched by a partner is that it is difficult to adjust the force of the stretch, since your partner cannot feel any pain you may experience, and could easily overstretch you. The concept of warm up, which I described earlier, applies very much to muscle stretching. You should have a really good warm up of the muscles concerned, and begin the stretching exercises very gradually.

In one sense, you are very fortunate to be mobilising your joints at the right age. In fact, most young children up to the age of four or five have extremely flexible joints. The simplest thing is to *maintain* this flexibility through childhood and youth, but most children don't bother with mobilising exercise unless they happen to be dancers or gymnasts. They lose all this suppleness, and by the time they reach their late teens are so stiff that they can't even do the latest dances.

Cheating

Most body movements involve more than one joint, sometimes a dozen or more joints are involved. The human body is a crafty machine, and will generally select the easiest method of performing whatever activity you ask of it. This is especially true in suppleness, when a relatively stiff joint will be given very little to do, leaving more flexible joints to perform most of the movement. This is called cheating, and can be overcome by isolating the stiff joint from the others, then working it on its own. The resulting movement may not be very great, but it can be extremely useful.

Exercises

In one sense there are no limits to the amount of stretching exercise that you may do. Muscles and ligaments don't get 'tired' in the normal sense by stretching. So it's very much a case of 'suck it and see', judging from the results of your exercises just how much you need to do.

Work out for yourself, or get some advice on, how much suppleness you need both for general life and also for any specific activities you may wish to do. My own advice is to base your exercises on whole movements rather than individual joints, remembering my earlier remarks about cheating. So, if you want to be able to bend over and weed the garden without aches and pains, then that is exactly the movement you should do. If it's mobile hips and spine that you want, so that you can better do your own thing at the disco, then the movements you have to exercise are much more complex – and may need to be broken down to the individual joints. Whatever you do, remember to take it easy at first. The principles of overload still apply in training for suppleness.

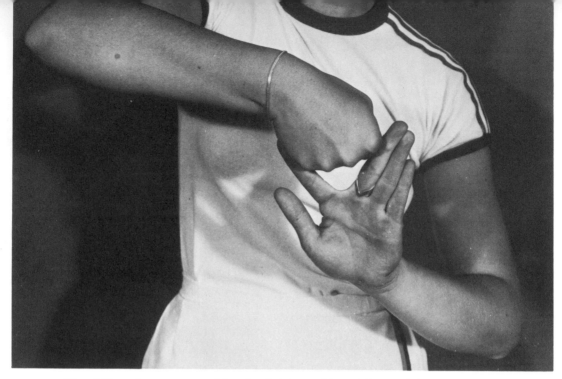

Hand Exercises   pushing back joints of knuckles and fingers, using other hand, or pushing against flat surface. Basketballers need to develop their finger suppleness to achieve better ball control.

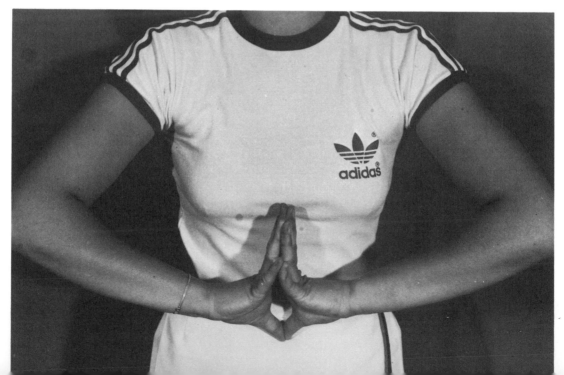

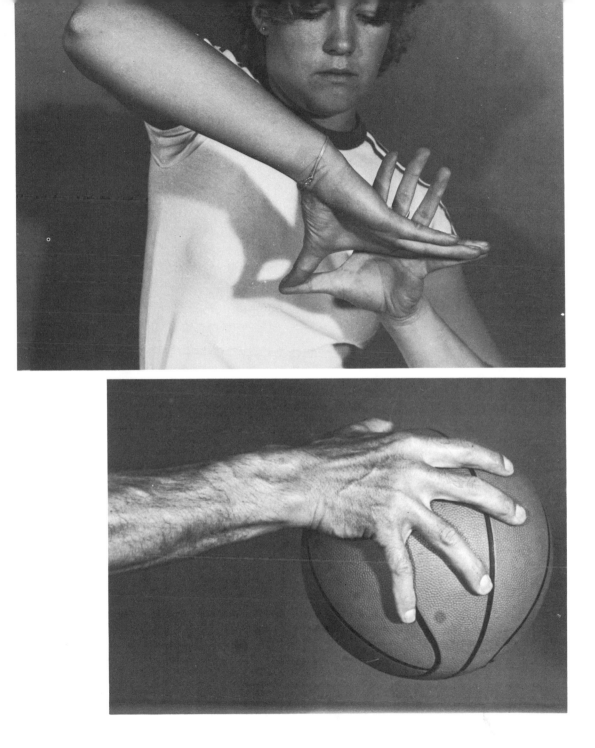

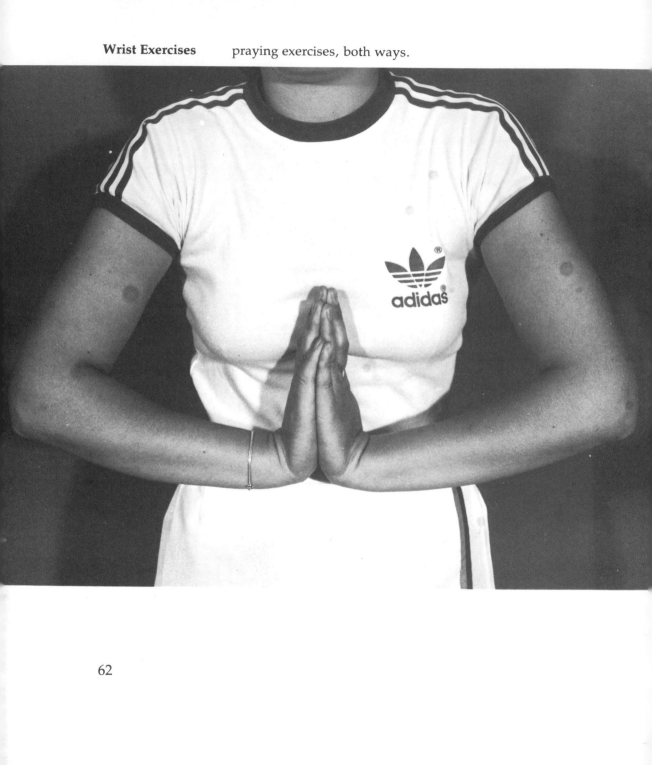

62

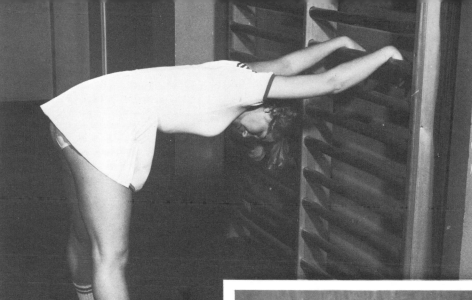

Shoulder Exercises
shoulder elevation – standing, hands
on wall – or kneeling, hands on
chair. Back scratching, both hands.

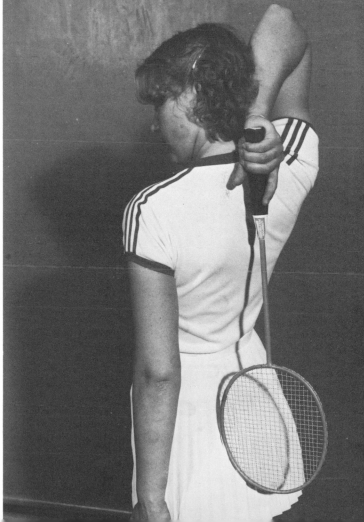

Back Exercises
prone, head and shoulder raise. Hang over back of chair or bench (see pages 46–7). Crabs, various. Be extra careful on these exercises.

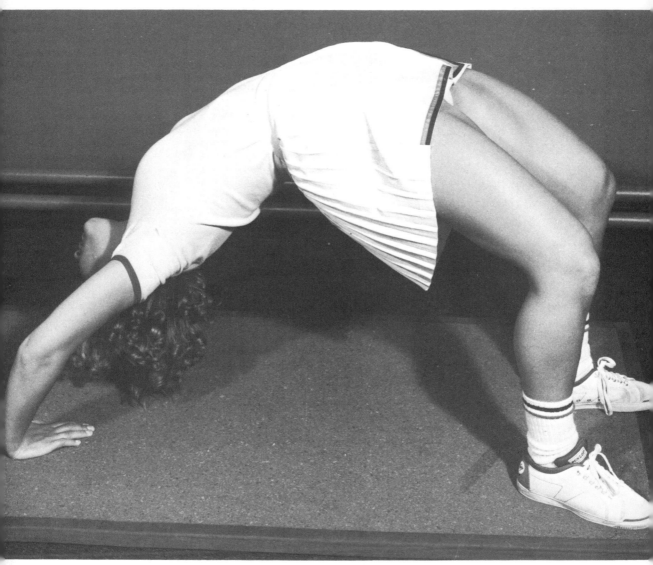

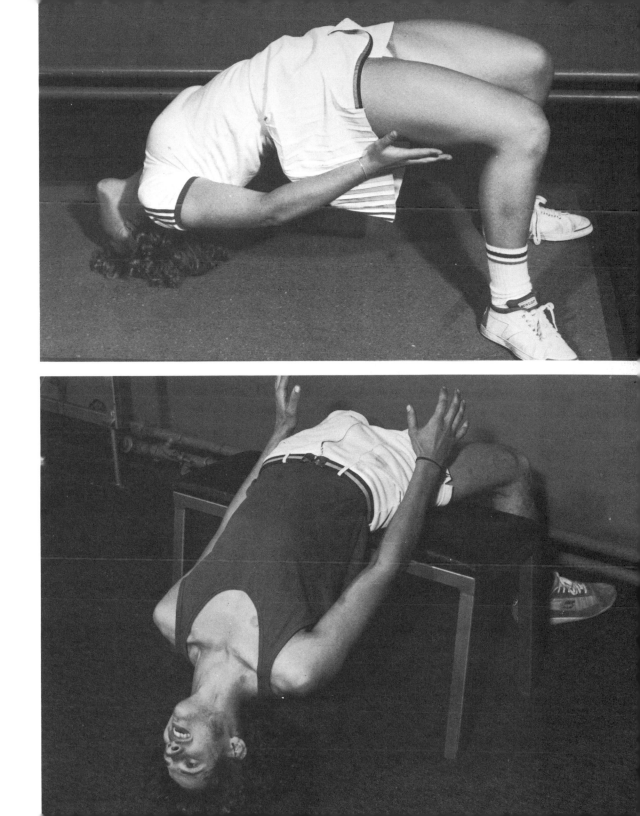

Waist Exercises kneel or sit, drops and twists, either side. Try to keep the hips facing front.

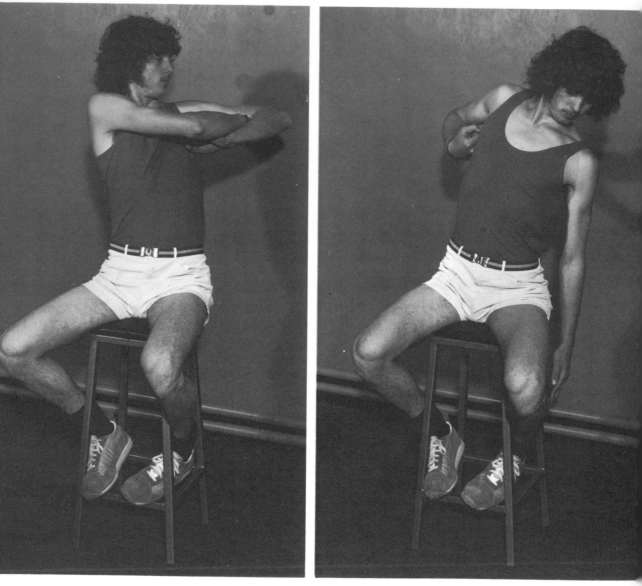

Hip Exercises lying leg raises, hurdling, yoga, splits, hip rolling, toes touching. It's easy to make up your own.

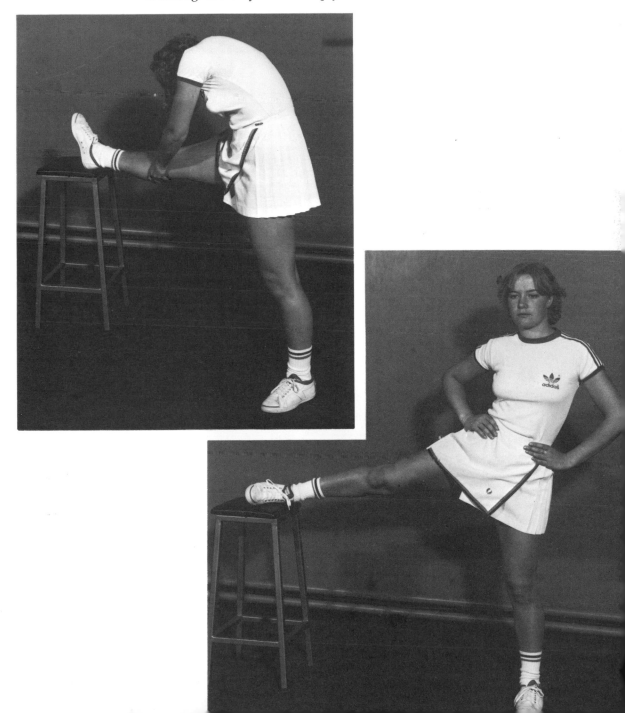

Ankle Exercises rolling, incline or ramp. Prone lying toes pointing. Make sure to stress in all directions necessary.

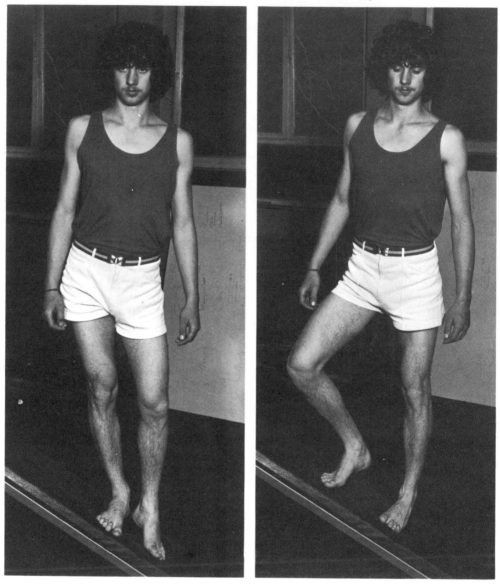

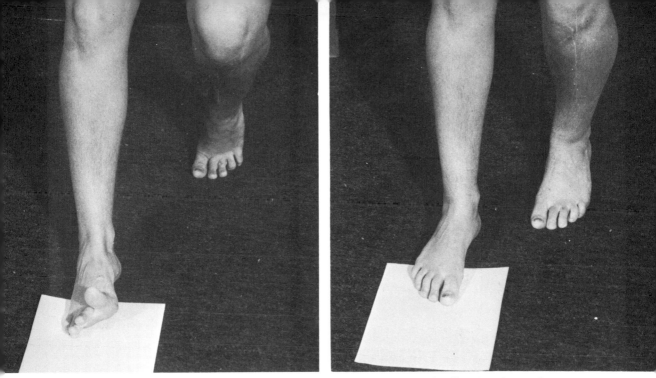

Foot Exercises   piano exercises. Spreading. High arching (pulling a piece of paper along the floor while keeping the heel still). Picking up objects. Your toes will cramp quite easily at first, but keep at it as soon as they recover.

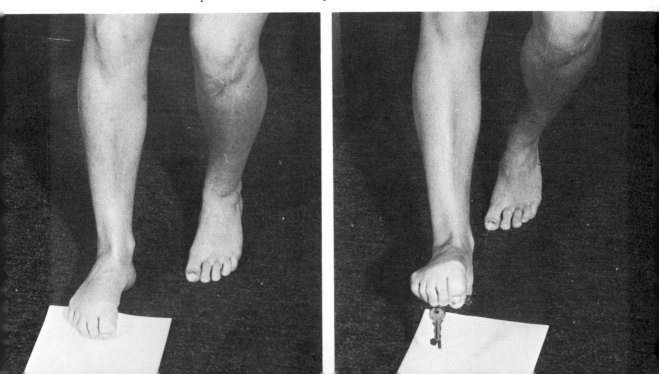

Testing Your Suppleness

It is very difficult to get an accurate measure of suppleness. Each person is so different in the way their joints interact that standard tests are almost meaningless. Your best bet is just to measure your own performance at the exercises you do. For example, on the straight leg toe touching you might be so stiff when you begin that you can only just touch your ankles. Then you keep going until one day you can touch the floor with your finger tips, then your palms. Eventually you will be able to touch your knees with your head. I doubt that you will want any more flexibility than that.

5. Speed

There are many different kinds of fitness which are called speed. For instance, you need speed to play snap, to play fast guitar music, to beat an opponent to the ball in soccer, to throw a javelin a long way, to hit a table tennis ball hard, to do a somersault – and yet each type of speed is different from the others!

Let's break it down. Basically, speed involves the idea of time – getting something done in a short space of time. What has to be done in that short space of time can involve the brain, the nerves, and the muscles. Training for speed has to concentrate on these three.

The Brain

Most of the functions of your brain are carried out without you being aware of it. Conscious thought is normally reserved for the things which are not habit, things you are not accustomed to. For example, you may eat a meal without being very aware of all the actions you make in loading your fork, putting it in your mouth, removing the food from the fork, chewing and swallowing it. You could be watching television, reading or talking at the time, leaving your automatic brain to sort out for you all the little difficulties of eating.

Many of the actions you perform can be speeded up if you train yourself to do them automatically; but you must be very sure that you want them to become automatic, because once you have trained yourself in this way, it is very difficult to prevent an automatic response on the odd occasion when it would be the wrong thing to do. If, for instance, you have trained yourself to very speedily and automatically swerve to the left if anyone gets in the way when you are driving – and then it happens on a mountain road with a 100 feet drop on your left, you could have a very short period in which to regret your training.

There are, of course, some very important conscious things the brain has to do as quickly as possible. These are situations where the brain has to examine the situation very carefully, and decide on one of several courses of action. A basketball player may have the options of passing to any one of his four team-mates, or shooting, or holding on to the ball and waiting for a better opportunity. He has a fraction of a second in which to make up his mind. These are very difficult decisions.

What many people do not realise is that the brain can be trained to greater speed in decision making. Firstly, it can learn the techniques of handling all the information quickly. Secondly, it can develop the ability to reason quickly. People who have fit brains can reach decisions much more quickly than others.

The Nerves

The nerves are like wires along which messages pass. The speed at which the messages travel seems to be fixed for each individual, and there is really nothing you can do in training to alter that speed. What you can do however is to shorten the distance the messages travel, by bypassing some of the nervous system. This is done by training your reflexes.

Reflex actions are generally over and done with before you know it, or even *without* you knowing it. If you touch a hot plate, you start to remove your hand before the brain becomes aware of the pain. If a fly heads towards your eye, you will usually blink before you are aware of seeing it. Many of these reflexes are in you at birth, but with careful repetitive training you can adapt them or even develop new ones.

The Muscles

Sooner or later, the muscle gets the message from the nerves telling it to act. Two things affect the speed of its reaction to this message.

The first thing is the *readiness* of the muscle, sometimes called the tone or tension of the muscle. If a muscle is 'on its mark', so to speak, waiting to explode into action when the signal comes, then it will react very quickly. This tone can be developed by training – in fact the strength training mentioned in chapter 3 will develop muscle tone – and also by mental preparation at the time the movement is needed.

The second thing is the muscle's power, that is a combination of the strength of the muscle and rate at which the strength can be used. Some people may be very strong, but slow and clumsy in the use of their strength. Such people are not very powerful, whereas others who may not have such great strength can use it quickly and therefore powerfully.

This brings us to something which is not very well understood by people trying to get fit. It is called the 'power to weight ratio'. Put in an uncomplicated way, it means that the speed you are going to be able to achieve will depend on achieving great power while keeping the weight being moved (the resistance) to a minimum.

The mechanical laws which govern this relationship are quite complex, and their interpretation is dependent on whether the object to be speeded up is your own body, or not. Where you are trying to move your own body quickly – such as running, rowing, jumping, tumbling, swimming – there comes a point where the extra weight put on when you build up muscle overtakes the extra power gained from the muscle.

On the other hand, when you are building up speed in some external heavy object (like shot or hammer, or opponent in rugby) then an increase in your own weight can be a decided advantage. Since the resistance against which you are working does *not* increase as you become more powerful, then your power to weight ratio improves. This is why all world champions in heavy resistance sports are very big heavy men.

There is a third category where, though the resistance is external, it is a very light one. Such resistances can be moved very speedily – such as a shuttlecock, tennis ball, golf ball – and the most important thing is the speed you can build up in your arms which is then transferred by a racquet. In this case, very large and powerful muscles may not be of much use. It must be borne in mind that the resistance to your power might be increased by inefficient movements. A swimmer with an inefficient stroke creates enormous water resistances, whereas a good swimmer seems to glide through the water most easily.

The Two R's

We can now take a look at the important differences between the two R's – reflexes, and reactions. You will frequently hear the words reflex and reaction used as if they meant the same, but the early parts of this chapter will have shown you that although a reflex action *is* a reaction to some stimulus or other, reactions which involves conscious thought are *not* reflexes. In reaction training it is vital to improve the operations of the brain, whereas in reflex training the aim is to do away with the part played by the brain altogether.

Speed versus Accuracy

Very frequently, people who are learning to do something accurately *and* quickly are faced with a problem of priority in training. This is true whether the activity is table tennis or typing, playing golf or guitar, sewing or skiing.

The problem is that the actual movements used when doing the activity at a slow speed are often very different from those used doing the activity at high speed. So if you learn at one speed, you may break down at another. But if you try to achieve high speed first, the movement may be totally wrong, which would be even worse.

The answer in this case seems to be a combination of the two. Whilst it would be wrong, for example, to try to play music quickly before the correct fingering had been learned – as soon as the fingering is correct the player ought to increase his speed, concentrating on both the development of accuracy and speed simultaneously.

Exercises

Remembering that the development of a good power to weight ratio involves building strength, and perhaps reducing weight, we should divide our speed exercises into those which affect brain, nerves and muscles.

Muscle

When training the muscles for speed, the exercises must be done *at* speed, or very powerfully. The first thing to be borne in mind is that the body must be thoroughly warmed up before starting speed training – these are the sessions where injury is most likely.

You must carefully select the movements you want to be speeded up. Sprint running training is of no use to a concert pianist! If a movement is a very complicated one, you may want to split it down into more easily manageable parts. This can be dangerous if by doing so you change the movement at all, or disturb the balance between the parts.

You must now structure a speed training session which includes periods of low resistance training where there can be several dozen repetitions of the movement at a faster than normal pace. Perhaps sprinting over 20 or 30 yards, bowling a lighter ball, cycling on a lower gear, or whatever.

Then there should be a similar time devoted to power training, against a slightly higher resistance than normal – maybe 10 or 20% higher. You should try to move just as quickly against this increased resistance, in a very explosive manner. If the resistance is too great, it becomes mere strength training which is valuable for other reasons described earlier. Examples of power training are: sprinting with a resistance such as a high geared bike, a drogue in swimming, uphill or wearing a weighted belt; putting a heavier shot, playing basketball with a medicine ball, boxing with heavy gloves, etc. etc.

The speed training session should also contain a substantial part devoted to the 'real thing', that is the movement performed at maximum speed against normal resistance. You should concentrate on moving efficiently with good style, trying to 'flow' at very high speed.

74

Nerves

Again, selecting carefully the movements to be trained, you must be sure that accuracy of movement is maintained. Then, work out what the signal is, to which you want to develop a reflex. It could be the gun in a sprint start, a straight left from a boxer, a lunge in fencing. From that moment on, the only secret is 'accelerating repetition'. That means that the signal should be given, followed by the accurate movement. The interval between the signal and the response should gradually be made shorter, maintaining the accuracy of each.

After many thousands of repetitions, you will find that your response will become a reflex. Let's hope you choose the right response in the first place!

Brain

This is a very misunderstood area of speed training. Remember that in this case we are not trying to develop reflexes, but rather the ability to process information quickly and come to the right decision. The first and perhaps most important technique is to be able to extract the important information from the bewildering variety of information available. Only a few small facts may be necessary, particularly if you are trying to predict what is about to happen.

Let's take it that you are riding a bike along a busy town road. You can see all the people walking about, the cars and buses driving past you, the skid patches of wet shiny road, the traffic lights up ahead, the window displays in the shops, the weather conditions, etc. You can hear the various noises made by all these, as well as the sound of a train passing by, a factory hooter, an airplane overhead, and so on. Additionally you can feel the saddle, the handlebars, the road surface through the tyres – and finally you can smell the exhaust fumes, the new baked bread, the coffee shop and the hops from the brewery.

Some of these pieces of information may be stored by you to be recalled later – the smells, some of the sounds, some of the sights. Other pieces may be rejected as unimportant, like an uninteresting window display or the sound of an aircraft. Some information will immediately be processed for short term action, e.g. how are the traffic lights changing – can I make it in time or should I slow down now? Other information may not be easily obtained, but must be looked for if you are to be able to react quickly. Is there a dog loose on the pavement, a pedestrian near a crossing, a parked car with children around? If so, then you must predict the next likely signal – that is, the dog darting into the road, the pedestrian suddenly claiming his right of way, a child chasing a ball from behind the car – and prepare for the response.

Sometimes I smile when I hear complimentary comments about some sports star's fantastic 'reflexes'. I know that it is humanly impossible to achieve reflex action times as quick as some players appear to do. It is just that they have trained themselves to extract the relevant information in sufficient time to begin their response very early. A squash pro doesn't wait until he sees which direction the ball is hit by his opponent before moving to the next shot. He watches his opponent prepare for the stroke, then watches the way the racquet head moves. By that time, he knows where the ball is going to go, and can begin his response. Yet, a beginner might not even watch his opponent play the stroke, and not see the ball until it is coming back at him off the front wall.

The second part of brain training is to learn what are the possible alternative actions from which you must select, and to practise the selection of the right one for each situation. This can be a very complicated process, and is generally better done under the supervision of a coach or with the help of friends.

There must be literally millions of such situations, and no way that I can suggest specific exercises to you. So, let's just have one example!

A midfield footballer in possession faces a complex defensive and attacking set up. The opposition apply an offside trap at every opportunity. A Striker wants a lead pass, behind the defence, on to which he can sprint clear of his defender. The striker makes a quick move back towards his own goal which simultaneously lulls his defender into following him, and gives the signal to the midfield player to make the pass immediately. The striker then changes direction and accelerates hard on to the ball, thus defeating the offside trap. The midfield player must be trained to look for such signals, and respond quickly with the right action, i.e. an accurate pass, because any delay in making the pass means a lost possession for 'offside'. That training should involve a gradual increase in the number of repetitions of the complete situation, and also a gradual introduction of other information which tends to distract the passer of the ball.

Tests of Speed

You will realise that this is a very difficult area for testing. Things like sprinting speed can of course be measured quite easily, especially in competition. Reaction time can also be measured using simple electronic equipment – if you can get hold of it! But brain function time is almost impossible for you to measure, and maybe you are just going to have to assess your improvement by how quickly you feel you perform in the real situation.

Anyway, there are a couple of tests in chapter 7. See how you get on with these!

6. Stamina

Stamina means the ability to 'keep going'. Even the easiest of movements, like placing one foot in front of the other, requires stamina if you are going to do it more than once. Not much stamina, it's true, but if you have to do it 50,000 times in one go – like a world championship race walker – then it needs superlative stamina just to complete the distance let alone doing it at about 7½ mph (about twice normal walking pace).

Of all the fitness elements we have looked at, stamina is the most complicated. We don't even know whether it means not getting tired, or not letting the feelings of tiredness slow us down. We can't even sort out whether tiredness refers to the actual state of the muscles, or just the way the muscle feels. Stamina may involve the ability to concentrate for long periods of time, or the ability to perform a heavy movement twice in succession. It's not surprising that so few people really understand it.

So, let us divide stamina into various categories, and we may then avoid confusion!

The author, 445 – who beat the world record for 25 miles race walking.

Muscle

When a muscle works, rather like an engine it requires fuel and oxygen to provide the energy. There are exhaust products, which you would expect – an acid called lactic acid which hangs around until it can be changed back into fuel, and carbon dioxide gas which gets blown away in your breath. The muscle carries its own small store of fuel, more is contained in the blood, and a large amount is stored in various parts of the body. The blood also receives oxygen from the air you breathe, and carries it to the muscles.

The stamina of a muscle must depend, therefore, on the amount of fuel it has in its own stores, and how much fuel and oxygen can be delivered by the blood, pumped by the heart. The first one is the one we call muscle stamina, or sometimes muscle endurance.

Circulation

The second stamina is called core endurance, or general stamina. This involves the function of lungs, heart and blood vessels. These ensure that enough blood, rich in fuel and oxygen, can get to any group of muscles which needs it.

Mental

Some activities which go on a long time – like games, wallpaper hanging, marathon running – require you to keep concentrating on the activity otherwise performance suffers. This is an enormously difficult thing for the mind to do, and requires to be specially trained.

Efficiency

Again, rather like a bike or car, you need to move efficiently. If your actions are stiff or clumsy, then your fuel consumption goes up – which means you run out of fuel earlier. When you have to do a movement only once or twice at a time, you might get away with inefficiency. When you have to do it a thousand times or more, even a little inefficiency can become intolerable.

Pain Tolerance

Fatigue hurts! It can hurt in many ways, but whatever the pain your commonsense tells you to stop the activity, and lie down until the pain goes away. The development of stamina includes the building up of your tolerance of pain, so that you can grit your teeth and bear it, or even make the pain disappear by willpower.

Recovery

Stamina includes the ability to recover quickly from fatigue. A weightlifter gets the bar to his shoulders on the first movement, then pauses for a second or two in order to recover, then completes the lift on the second move. A gardener digs out a heavy spadeful, rests for a few seconds then digs another, and so on. Most amazingly of all the heart muscle squeezes out the blood, recovers for only a fraction of a second, and beats again, and again, maintaining this non stop for the whole of your life!

Recovery tends to be divided into full and partial. Full recovery occurs when you are able to rest for long enough to fully recover before working again. Partial recovery describes resting periods where you can recover some or most of your strength, but have to work again before fully recovered. If you keep going for a long time with only partial recovery periods, your tiredness keeps building up until you are forced to stop or slow down.

Training for Stamina

All training is based on overload, and stamina is no exception. But we must work out what kind of stamina we need, and plan our training schedule to meet these needs.

Muscle Training. This is achieved by reducing the load against which the muscle is working, and performing perhaps two or three times the number of repetitions. For a weightlifter that will mean only two or three reps, at a slightly lower weight – for a miler that might mean two miles at a slightly slower pace.

Depending on the activity, you could do anything from two to perhaps twenty sets of those reps – a lower number of sets for the longer duration activity. Remember also that you must do your activity efficiently, cutting out wasteful movements.

General Stamina Training. There are two forms of this, continuous and interval. In continuous training it's unbroken quantity that counts. Cyclists call this 'getting the miles in'. The rate at which you are working should only be about 60% of your maximum, but you should quite literally keep it going for ages. It you are training for cycling, running, walking, canoeing or anything like that, a continuous general endurance session can go on for hours – *but work up to it gradually, and maintain efficient action.*

79

Interval training involves working for short periods at a *greater* load than normal with short rest periods in between each burst of activity. This develops recovery stamina. It can be done very informally, like going on a cross country run and stopping every so often to admire the view, do exercises or get your breath back. This method is called Fartlek.

Or you can be more formal by training with a partner, with one working – say, for a minute – while the other rests, and then changing over. This is called Paarlauf, and can be kept going for as much as an hour. It can also be done as a continuous relay race.

The most complicated form of interval training involves working out exactly how much work, and how much rest, and how many repetitions, and how many sets you are going to do. Schedules vary between different types and lengths of activity being trained for, and between different people. Here is an example of a running interval training schedule for a good standard athlete; lasting one hour and a half.

Warm Up – 10 minutes
Set 1   – 4 laps of 400m. in 65 secs, 1 minute rest between each.
                Rest for 10 minutes (walking and jogging)
Set 2   – 8 × 200m. at 30 secs, 1 minute rest between each.
                Rest for 10 minutes (walking and jogging)
Set 3   – 5 × 100m. at 14 secs, 30 seconds rest between each.
                Rest 10 minutes (walking and jogging)
Set 4   – 5 × 30 secs shuttleruns at top speed, 15 seconds
                rest between each.
                Rest for 10 minutes (walking)
Run one mile at medium pace.

Now, this would be a very demanding session for a senior athlete. You would need to scale it down, both in toughness and length, to suit your own requirements. You really should get a P.E. teacher or coach to advise you, and remember – work up to it gently!

Circuit Training

This is a very special form of training which concentrates on pain tolerance and general endurance, while still giving an all round muscle training as well. I have no hesitation in telling you that it is by far the best form of general fitness training, from almost any point of view.

The idea is that you select six or eight strength exercises, perhaps some that I have shown you in chapter 3. There should be two or three of leg exercises, one stomach and one back exercise, two or three arm bending and stretching exercises, and a shoulder exercise. They should be organised so that as you do each exercise in its turn you go from leg to trunk to arm to leg to trunk, and so on. This allows you to work flat out on each muscle group and then rest it while other groups are having their turn. Once through all the exercises is called a Circuit.

Now, although we let each muscle rest in turn, the important thing is not to let the heart and lungs recover. You must go straight from one exercise to the next without stopping, and you must keep each exercise going as fast as you can until the time to change.

There are different ways of organising circuit training, but if more than one person at a time is doing it, someone should act as leader. The equipment (if any) that you are using should all be laid out ready, and you shouldn't have to fiddle around with it when you get to it. At each exercise you should either have a target number of repetitions, or a set time to complete. If target reps, then you must do them as quickly as possible. If set time, then you must do as many reps as possible in that time.

The most efficient way of organising the equipment is by using a multistation exercise machine.

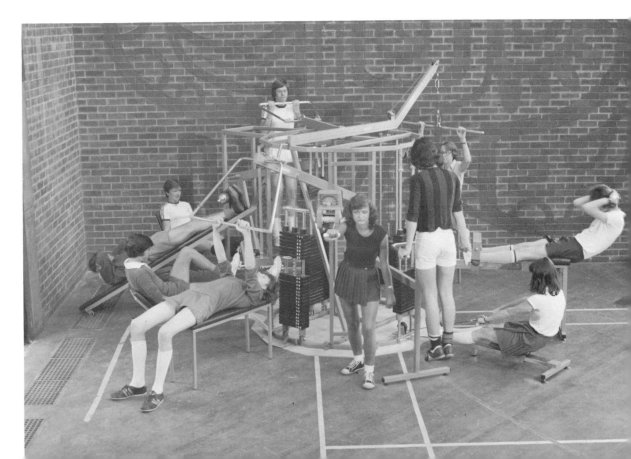

If a group of you are circuit training together, then the set time method is best, with the leader calling out 'Change' every 30, 45 or 60 seconds (depending which of those you select). He must obviously be able to see a sweep second hand, or a digital clock.

If on your own, then the target repetition method is best because you don't have to worry about the time.

As you get fitter, you can increase the reps, increase the loads, increase the times, and increase the number of circuits. Again, I must advise you to work up to it gradually. Nothing is more demanding than a really hard circuit training session.

Tests of Stamina

Many good tests of stamina have been developed, and I have included some in chapter 7. On the other hand, your own performance in stamina training is easy to measure, and can give you the information you need about your own improvement.

7. Where do you go from here?

If you have read straight through this book, you have probably got some idea of the general approach to 'better fitness'. On the other hand, there is rather a lot of information crammed into a small space, and you would need to be a genius to go straight out and put everything into operation. So, where *do* you go from here?

1. The first thing is to decide whether you really do want to be fit. Fitness training as such is not something many people would chose to do just for the fun of it. You would be better off playing some games or taking up some hobbies, if fun is all you want. No, the fun comes when you do all these other things better, *because* you are fitter.

2. The second thing is to work out carefully the things you want to be fit for. Put together a 'shopping list' of fitness goodies:

  1oz of strong heart
  4lb of arm muscles
  10lb of leg muscle
  5° of shoulder extension etc. etc. (I'm joking, really!! You can't really measure these things like butter and eggs.)

3. Then you should test your fitness, using the kinds of test mentioned later in this chapter – or others which may appeal to you. This gives you a base line, against which you can gauge your progress.

4. Now work out your targets, maybe for a period of a year. These may not be very realistic aims, and you may have to revise them later. Your experiences during the early stages will show you whether you are training too often or too seldom, whether you are under or over ambitious, and so on. But, having long term aims will keep in your mind that the benefits are long term, and prevent you from becoming too easily satisfied with your progress.

5. At this stage, you are ready to organise your training. Following the guidelines mentioned in chapter 2 make sure that, as far as is possible, bad organisation is not going to reduce the benefits of your training efforts. Included in this should be the preparation of record books, training diaries, progress graphs or any other form of

record. I always prefer graphs myself, and I stick them on the wall where I can see them often. This gives me a lot of pleasure and motivation, but also interests other people who tend to follow my example!

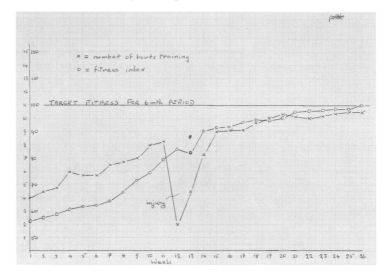

Advice

The last thing to do before starting is to take some specialist advice. You don't have to pay the earth for this – in fact you can usually get it for nothing. One very important point is your medical condition. If you are a very fat person, or if there is any record of heart problems in your family, then you should see your doctor to make sure that you don't have a defective heart. Other medical conditions, particularly things like diabetes and epilepsy, may also effect your exercise program. That is not to say that any medical condition should stop you doing exercise. On the contrary, exercise is virtually the universal medicine, provided that it is taken in the proper 'doses'. But in these cases, medical advice is always a *must*.

Another necessary source of advice is P.E. teachers. They have been specially trained in many things mentioned in this book. Whilst it is not usually practical for them to give *everyone* the individual attention they really need, if you show interest in your own fitness – especially by planning your own training schedules and measuring your own fitness – I can't imagine many teachers ignoring your request.

Several other professions are knowledgeable about the effects of exercise. These

84

include physiotherapists, remedial gymnasts, sport coaches and osteopaths. But, don't be surprised if you occasionally get conflicting advice. Not everything is hard and fast, and different professions are trained for different purposes and in different ways. There are many different paths which arrive at the same place.

The last source of advice I should mention is books. The fact that you are reading these words shows that you are prepared to take advice from a book. It has not been possible for me to go into great detail on many of the points I have mentioned, otherwise this book would have been huge – and expensive. So, I shall mention a few books to which you can refer if you are interested in knowing more.

Title	Publishers	Author	Contents
Science & Sport	Faber & Faber	Thomas	General scientific basis of training and sport. Simple
Circuit Training	Bell & Hyman	Morgan & Adamson	Full description of circuit training methods
Aerobics	Bantam Books	Cooper	Simple methods of general exercising and self testing
Exercise Physiology	Playball Promotions	Thomas	Very technical coverage of the whole subject
Introduction to Tests and Measurements in P.E.	Bell	Campbell & Tucker	General text on fitness testing

Fitness Clubs

Many people prefer to train for fitness in groups. Of course, this can be done by forming your own group at school, or amongst your friends. Another way is to join a club, which not only helps to keep you highly motivated and well organised, but also brings social benefits which add to the value of your training. Many sports clubs have organised training which is very beneficial, but it is usually specific to the sport practised in that club. Clubs which have been formed mainly for fitness training are relatively few, but are currently increasing rapidly in number. They are generally organised within educational programs, either at school, college or evening institutes. Indeed, you could form one at your own school.

Another area of development has been in public sport and leisure centres. Many of these have excellent fitness training facilities, and some run fitness clubs. If a club doesn't exist, then ask the centre management to form one.

One final suggestion is that you look to youth organisations which might provide club facilities or classes. Organisations such as Y.M.C.A., Y.W.C.A., Youth Clubs, National Association of Boys Clubs, etc., have a long history of such activities.

Tests

In earlier chapters I have explained how difficult it is to test some fitness elements, and how easy to test others. Also there is the problem that in some cases, your own performance can be compared quite accurately with the performance of others of your own age and sex, whereas in other cases you can only really compare yourself with your own standard some time ago. Whatever is the case, and all methods are useful to you in assessing your state of fitness, you must realise that a test is only as accurate as *you* make it. Accurate measurement of length would be difficult if your ruler was made of elastic, or if you used the centimetre scale one time and the inch scale the next – without knowing the difference.

You can only compare accurately if you do the tests absolutely properly, fulfilling the conditions of the test to the letter, and doing it the same way each time. It is usually helpful if someone else supervises the tests, who can make an unbiased judgement of your performance. People have been known to cheat themselves in fitness testing! Though I am sure that you wouldn't cheat knowingly, it is still possible to do it unknowingly.

I have chosen from amongst the dozens of recognised international tests, since they are not only good ones but also there are 'normal scores' against which you can compare yourself. But remember, they are only a rough guide, and there might be all sorts of reasons for you to be much better or worse than average, including that you might just be having an offday for some reason. Personally, I like to make up my own tests to measure my own progress, so why not do that too?

Chins

This is a test of arm and shoulder, involving strength and muscle endurance. Hang at full stretch from a bar about 1½ ins thick, using an overgrasp. The bar should be high enough for your feet to clear the ground. Pull up until your chin can clear the bar, then lower yourself until your arms are straight again. You should not jerk, or kick your legs around, or sway your body. Count one point every time your chin actually clears the bar. No half points, no allowances for 'almost there'. See page 28.

For girls, the bar should be fixed at breast height, with the feet placed forward and on the floor, and with the body straight to such an extent that the arms form a right angle with the body. Or, achieve the same position by resting the feet on a box or stool. Use rubber soles or a mat to prevent the feet from sliding.

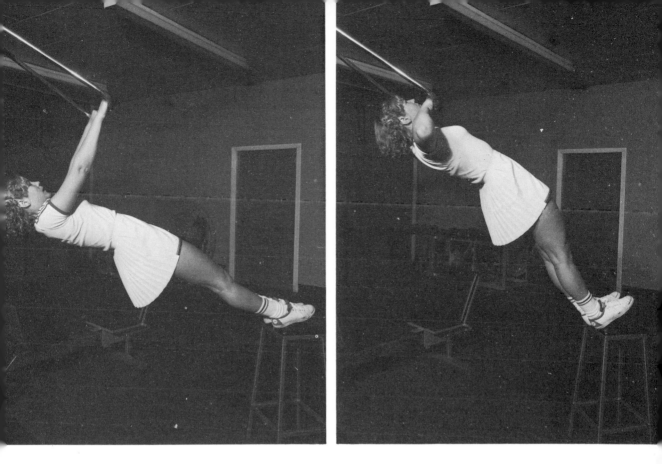

SCORES

<table>
<tr><td colspan="9" align="center">BOYS</td><td colspan="8" align="center">GIRLS</td></tr>
<tr><td>Age</td><td>10</td><td>11</td><td>12</td><td>13</td><td>14</td><td>15</td><td>16</td><td>17</td><td>10</td><td>11</td><td>12</td><td>13</td><td>14</td><td>15</td><td>16</td><td>17</td></tr>
<tr><td>Excellent</td><td>9</td><td>8</td><td>7</td><td>7</td><td>8</td><td>9</td><td>9</td><td>10</td><td>40</td><td>50</td><td>60</td><td>60</td><td>60</td><td>60</td><td>50</td><td>40</td></tr>
<tr><td>Good</td><td>6</td><td>5</td><td>4</td><td>4</td><td>5</td><td>6</td><td>7</td><td>8</td><td>28</td><td>40</td><td>50</td><td>50</td><td>50</td><td>50</td><td>40</td><td>38</td></tr>
<tr><td>High Average</td><td>5</td><td>4</td><td>3</td><td>3</td><td>4</td><td>5</td><td>5</td><td>6</td><td>22</td><td>34</td><td>40</td><td>40</td><td>39</td><td>39</td><td>35</td><td>35</td></tr>
<tr><td>Low Average</td><td>3</td><td>3</td><td>2</td><td>3</td><td>3</td><td>4</td><td>4</td><td>5</td><td>15</td><td>22</td><td>32</td><td>32</td><td>32</td><td>32</td><td>30</td><td>30</td></tr>
<tr><td>Poor</td><td>2</td><td>2</td><td>2</td><td>2</td><td>2</td><td>3</td><td>3</td><td>3</td><td>12</td><td>12</td><td>22</td><td>20</td><td>20</td><td>22</td><td>24</td><td>25</td></tr>
<tr><td>Very Poor</td><td>1</td><td>1</td><td>1</td><td>1</td><td>1</td><td>2</td><td>2</td><td>2</td><td>8</td><td>6</td><td>10</td><td>10</td><td>9</td><td>14</td><td>19</td><td>22</td></tr>
</table>

Sit Ups

This is a test of abdominal muscle strength and endurance. You should lie on your back on a soft floor. Your legs must be straight, with your feet about one foot apart and secured by a bench, partner or heavy weight. Your hands should be clasped behind your head. You sit up, keeping your hands clasped and knees straight to touch one knee with the opposite elbow, then lie down again. That sit up scores one point. The next sit up should use the alternate elbow and knee. There is not much point going on if you can do more than 100 (for boys) or 50 (for girls) – you're too good for the test!

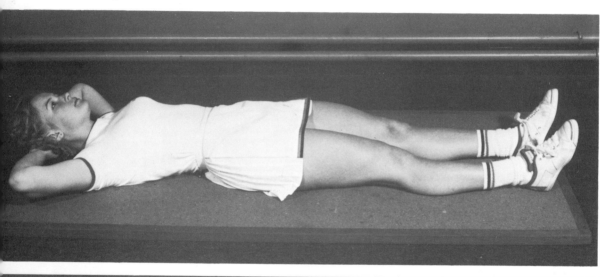

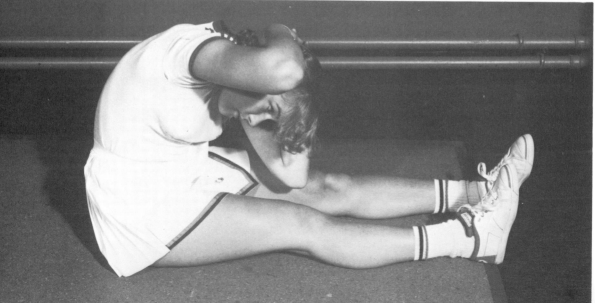

| | BOYS | | | | | | | | GIRLS | | | | | | | |
Age	10	11	12	13	14	15	16	17	10	11	12	13	14	15	16	17
Excellent	100	100	100	100	100	100	100	100	50	50	50	50	50	50	49	49
Good	55	58	63	70	77	70	59	55	39	43	47	48	39	37	39	39
High Average	41	44	48	51	55	52	50	47	30	34	36	37	31	28	31	32
Low Average	32	33	37	42	46	42	41	40	23	26	27	28	24	23	24	25
Poor	24	26	28	31	34	33	34	33	17	21	21	22	20	18	20	21
Very Poor	16	18	19	20	21	24	25	24	9	14	12	14	12	10	12	14

Shuttle Run

This is a test of speed and power, mainly of the legs. Two parallel lines should be marked on the floor, 30 feet apart. Starting behind one line, you run to put one foot beyond the other line, turn and run back to put one foot beyond the starting line, turn and run away again until you have run five times out and back. That equals 100 yards of running. Use a stop-watch, or a friend watching a sweep second hand and counting the seconds out loud. From the command 'Go' to crossing the finishing line should be timed to the nearest half second.

| | BOYS | | | | | | | | GIRLS | | | | | | | |
Age	10	11	12	13	14	15	16	17	10	11	12	13	14	15	16	17
Excellent	23	23.5	23.5	23	22.5	21.5	21	21	25.5	26	26	25.5	25	24	23.5	23.5
Good	25.5	26	26	25	25	25	24.5	24.5	28	28.5	28.5	27.5	27.5	27.5	26	26
High Average	26.6	27	27	26.5	26	26.5	25.5	25	29.5	30	30	29.5	29	29.5	28.5	28
Low Average	28	28.5	28.5	28	27.5	28	27	26	31	31.5	31.5	31	30.5	31	30	29
Poor	29	30	30	29	29.5	29.5	28.5	28	32.5	33.5	33.5	32.5	33	33	32	31.5
Very Poor	32	32.5	33	33	34	34	33	32	36	36.5	37	37	38	38	37	36

Vertical Jump

This is a test of all round power. Stand with your dominant side against a wall. Put chalk on your finger tips. Stretch up with the dominant hand and make a mark with your chalky fingers as high as you possibly can while keeping both feet flat on the

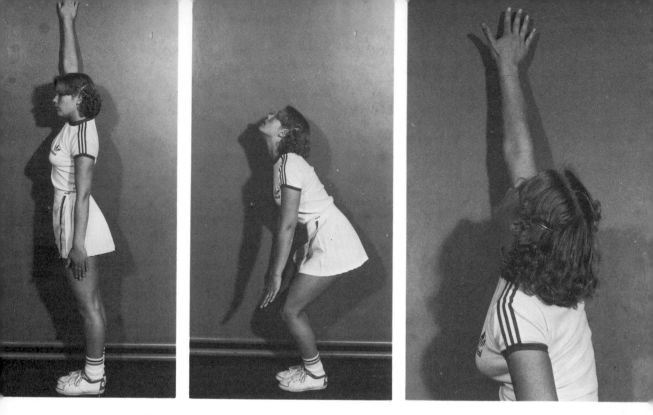

floor. Moving away from the wall a few inches, crouch ready to jump upwards. Without any preparatory swings or bounces, leap up to make a chalk finger mark as high as you possibly can. Then measure the distance between your standing mark and the highest mark, to the nearest half an inch. Repeat the test three times, and the highest jump is your score.

	BOYS								GIRLS							
Age	10	11	12	13	14	15	16	17	10	11	12	13	14	15	16	17
Excellent	15	17	19	20	21.5	22.5	23.5	24.5	12.5	14.5	16.5	17.5	19	20	21	22
Good		12.5	14.5	16	17.5	18.5	20	20.5	22	10.5	12.5	14	15.5	16.5	18	18.5	20
High Average	11.5	13	14.5	16	17	18	18.5	20	9.5	11	12.5	14	15	16	16.5	18
Low Average	10	11	13	14.5	15	16.5	17.5	19	8	9	11	12.5	13	14.5	15.5	17
Poor	9	9.5	11.5	12.5	13	15	15.5	17	7.5	8	10	11	11.5	13.5	14	15.5
Very Poor	6	6.5	7.5	9	10	12	13	14	5	5.5	6.5	8	9	11	12	13

600 yard run/walk

This is a test of running speed and medium general stamina. From a standing start, you run, or run and walk, 600 yards as fast as you can. Your time, in seconds, is your score.

	BOYS								GIRLS							
Age	10	11	12	13	14	15	16	17	10	11	12	13	14	15	16	17
Excellent	117	118	113	107	102	100	95	93	136	135	132	128	129	128	126	125
Good	129	125	121	116	111	107	102	99	148	146	143	141	139	138	136	135
High Average	135	131	125	121	117	111	106	102	157	153	152	148	146	148	146	144
Low Average	144	136	131	127	121	117	111	106	167	161	161	158	154	155	152	150
Poor	157	143	136	134	128	123	116	110	180	170	172	171	164	164	156	156
Very Poor	176	165	148	146	142	137	125	121	197	195	185	185	181	180	183	184

Step Test

This is the best test of general fitness of your heart. The test *must* be done very precisely, completely sticking to the laid down conditions. Stand facing a step, strong box or bench (18 ins high for boys, 16 ins high for girls). Either you or your friend, having a sweep second hand clearly in view, should call out a rhythm like this, 'up – and – down – and – up – and down – and ...' The 'up' occurs as the second hand passes one second mark. The 'down' occurs as the hand passes the next second mark. You will soon get the rhythm of the count going, especially if you keep your eye on the second hand (note – a metronome set to 120 beats per minute will do the job even better). In time with the rhythm you should step on to and off the box, standing perfectly upright with locked knees on the box. You can change your leading foot at any time if you want to, so long as you don't miss a step. You should keep this going, absolutely in time, for four minutes. If you can't keep up, by the time ten seconds of losing ground have passed you should stop. When you finish, sit down on the step immediately. Note how many seconds you managed to keep going, with a maximum of 240 if you completed the four minutes.

Find your pulse – which after exercise is most easily done at the neck – and count the number of beats in a 30 second period starting exactly one minute after stopping exercise. Make a note of the number of beats. Do the count again, starting

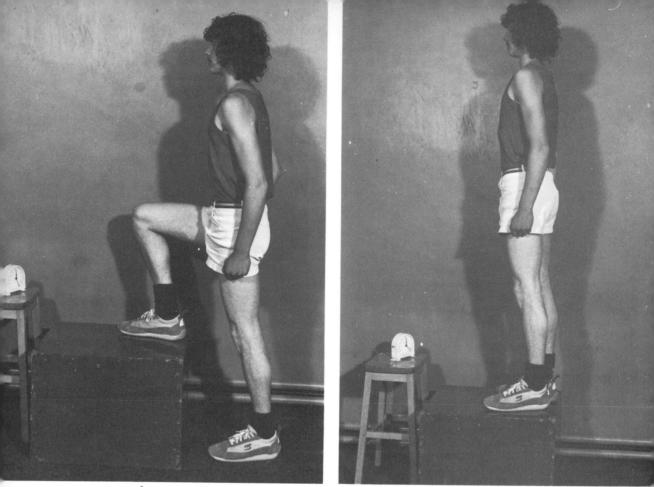

exactly two minutes after stopping exercise, and again at three minutes after stopping.

You now have four numbers. The first is the number of seconds you exercised for. The others are the three pulse counts, which should be added together to give a total pulse count. Your score is obtained from this simple formula:

$$\text{Endurance score} = \frac{\text{duration of exercise (in seconds)} \times 100}{2 \times \text{total pulse counts.}}$$

Shall we take an example. If you completed the four minutes, and had pulse counts of 75, 65 and 55, your score would be:

$$\frac{240 \times 100}{2 \times (75 + 65 + 55)} = 61.5$$

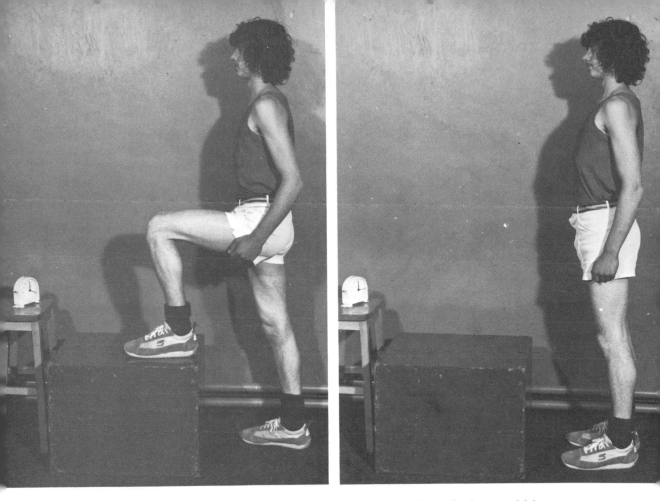

It is not possible to give you any other than a very rough idea of what could be expected of you on this test, and its best use is just to check your score as it changes with training. But, just for interest, here are some normal values which have been calculated for youngsters between 12 and 18 years old:

Superior   91 and over
Excellent   81–90
Good   71–80
Fair   61–70
Poor   51–60
Very Poor   50 and below.